THE YOGA OF DIVINE LOVE

THE SYNTHESIS OF YOGA

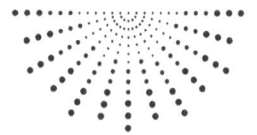

SRI AUROBINDO

CONTENTS

INTRODUCTION

Life and Yoga	3
The Three Steps of Nature	7
The Threefold Life	17
The Systems of Yoga	28
The Synthesis of the Systems	38

THE YOGA OF DIVINE LOVE

Love and the Triple Path	49
The Motives of Devotion	56
The Godward Emotions	65
The Way of Devotion	74
The Divine Personality	80
The Delight of the Divine	90
The Ananda Brahman	95
The Mystery of Love	101
Also by SRI AUROBINDO	109

INTRODUCTION

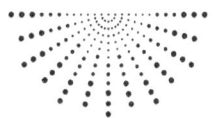

LIFE AND YOGA

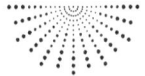

THERE are two necessities of Nature's workings which seem always to intervene in the greater forms of human activity, whether these belong to our ordinary fields of movement or seek those exceptional spheres and fulfilments which appear to us high and divine. Every such form tends towards a harmonised complexity and totality which again breaks apart into various channels of special effort and tendency, only to unite once more in a larger and more puissant synthesis. Secondly, development into forms is an imperative rule of effective manifestation; yet all truth and practice too strictly formulated becomes old and loses much, if not all, of its virtue; it must be constantly renovated by fresh streams of the spirit revivifying the dead or dying vehicle and changing it, if it is to acquire a new life. To be perpetually reborn is the condition of a material immortality. We are in an age, full of the throes of travail, when all forms of thought and activity that have in themselves any strong power of utility or any secret virtue of persistence are being subjected to a supreme test and given their opportunity of rebirth. The world today presents the aspect of a huge cauldron of Medea in which all things are being cast, shredded into pieces, experimented on, combined and recombined either to perish and provide the scattered material of new forms or to emerge rejuvenated and changed for a fresh term of existence. Indian

Yoga, in its essence a special action or formulation of certain great powers of Nature, itself specialised, divided and variously formulated, is potentially one of these dynamic elements of the future life of humanity. The child of immemorial ages, preserved by its vitality and truth into our modern times, it is now emerging from the secret schools and ascetic retreats in which it had taken refuge and is seeking its place in the future sum of living human powers and utilities. But it has first to rediscover itself, bring to the surface the profoundest reason of its being in that general truth and that unceasing aim of Nature which it represents, and find by virtue of this new self-knowledge and self-appreciation its own recovered and larger synthesis. Reorganising itself, it will enter more easily and powerfully into the reorganised life of the race which its processes claim to lead within into the most secret penetralia and upward to the highest altitudes of existence and personality.

In the right view both of life and of Yoga all life is either consciously or subconsciously a Yoga. For we mean by this term a methodised effort towards self-perfection by the expression of the secret potentialities latent in the being and—highest condition of victory in that effort—a union of the human individual with the universal and transcendent Existence we see partially expressed in man and in the Cosmos. But all life, when we look behind its appearances, is a vast Yoga of Nature who attempts in the conscious and the subconscious to realise her perfection in an ever-increasing expression of her yet unrealised potentialities and to unite herself with her own divine reality. In man, her thinker, she for the first time upon this Earth devises self-conscious means and willed arrangements of activity by which this great purpose may be more swiftly and puissantly attained. Yoga, as Swami Vivekananda has said, may be regarded as a means of compressing one's evolution into a single life or a few years or even a few months of bodily existence. A given system of Yoga, then, can be no more than a selection or a compression, into narrower but more energetic forms of intensity, of the general methods which are already being used loosely, largely, in a leisurely movement, with a profuser apparent waste of material and energy but with a more complete combination by the great Mother in her vast upward labour. It is this view of Yoga that can alone form the basis for a sound and rational synthesis of Yogic methods. For then Yoga ceases to appear something mystic and abnormal which has no relation to the ordinary processes of the World-Energy or the purpose she keeps in view in her two great movements of subjective and objective self-fulfilment; it reveals itself rather as an intense and exceptional use of powers that she has already manifested or is progressively organising in her less exalted but more general operations. Yogic methods have something of the same relation to the customary psychological workings of man as has the scientific handling of the force of electricity or of steam to their normal operations in Nature. And they, too, like the operations of Science, are formed upon a knowledge developed and confirmed by regular experiment, practical analysis and constant result. All Rajayoga, for instance, depends on this perception and experience that our inner elements, combinations, functions, forces, can be separated or dissolved, can be new-combined and set to novel and formerly impossible workings or can be transformed and resolved into a new general synthesis by fixed internal processes. Hathayoga similarly depends on this perception and experience that the vital forces and functions to which our life is normally subjected and whose ordinary operations seem set and indispensable, can be mastered and the operations changed or suspended with results that would otherwise be impossible and that seem miraculous to those who have not seized the rationale of their process. And if in some other of its forms this character of Yoga is less apparent, because they are more intuitive and less mechanical, nearer, like the Yoga of Devotion, to a supernal ecstasy or, like the Yoga of Knowledge, to a supernal infinity of consciousness and being, yet they too start from the use of some principal faculty in us by ways and for ends not contemplated in its everyday spontaneous workings. All methods grouped under the common name of Yoga are special psychological processes founded on a fixed truth of Nature and developing, out of normal functions, powers and results which were always latent but which her ordinary movements do not easily or do not often manifest.

But as in physical knowledge the multiplication of scientific processes has its disadvantages, as that tends, for instance, to develop a victorious artificiality which overwhelms our natural human life under a load of machinery and to purchase certain forms of freedom and mastery at the price of an increased servitude, so the preoccupation with Yogic processes and their exceptional results may have its disadvantages and losses. The Yogin tends to draw away from the common existence and lose his hold upon it; he tends to purchase wealth of spirit by an impoverishment of his human activities, the inner freedom by an outer death. If he gains God, he loses life, or if he turns his efforts outward to conquer life, he is in danger of losing God. Therefore we see in India that a sharp incompatibility has been created between life in the world and spiritual growth and perfection, and although the tradition and ideal of a victorious harmony between the inner attraction and the outer demand remains, it is little or else very imperfectly exemplified. In fact, when a man turns his vision and energy inward and enters on the path of Yoga, he is popularly supposed to be lost inevitably to the great stream of our collective existence and the secular effort of humanity. So strongly has the idea prevailed, so much has it been emphasised by prevalent philosophies and religions that to escape from life is now commonly considered as not only the necessary condition, but the general object of Yoga. No synthesis of Yoga can be satisfying which does not, in its aim, reunite God and Nature in a liberated and perfected human life or, in its method, not only permit but favour the harmony of our inner and outer activities and experiences in the divine consummation of both. For man is precisely that term and symbol of a higher Existence descended into the material world in which it is possible for the lower to transfigure itself and put on the nature of the higher and the higher to reveal itself in the forms of the lower. To avoid the life which is given him for the realisation of that possibility, can never be either the indispensable condition or the whole and ultimate object of his supreme endeavour or of his most powerful means of self-fulfilment. It can only be a temporary necessity under certain conditions or a specialised extreme effort imposed on the individual so as to prepare a greater general possibility for the race. The true and full object and utility of Yoga can only be accomplished when the conscious Yoga in man becomes, like the subconscious Yoga in Nature, outwardly conterminous with life itself and we can once more, looking out both on the path and the achievement, say in a more perfect and luminous sense:

"All life is Yoga."

THE THREE STEPS OF NATURE

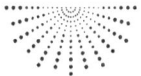

WE RECOGNISE then, in the past developments of Yoga, a specialising and separative tendency which, like all things in Nature, had its justifying and even imperative utility and we seek a synthesis of the specialised aims and methods which have, in consequence, come into being. But in order that we may be wisely guided in our effort, we must know, first, the general principle and purpose underlying this separative impulse and, next, the particular utilities upon which the method of each school of Yoga is founded. For the general principle we must interrogate the universal workings of Nature herself, recognising in her no merely specious and illusive activity of a distorting Maya, but the cosmic energy and working of God Himself in His universal being formulating and inspired by a vast, an infinite and yet a minutely selective Wisdom, *prajñā prasṛtā purāṇī* of the Upanishad, Wisdom that went forth from the Eternal since the beginning. For the particular utilities we must cast a penetrative eye on the different methods of Yoga and distinguish among the mass of their details the governing idea which they serve and the radical force which gives birth and energy to their processes of effectuation. Afterwards we may more easily find the one common principle and the one common power from which all derive their being and tendency, towards which all subconsciously move and in which, therefore, it is possible for all consciously to unite.

The progressive self-manifestation of Nature in man, termed in modern language his evolution, must necessarily depend upon three successive elements. There is that which is already evolved; there is that which, still imperfect, still partly fluid, is persistently in the stage of conscious evolution; and there is that which is to be evolved and may perhaps be already displayed, if not constantly, then occasionally or with some regularity of recurrence, in primary formations or in others more developed and, it may well be, even in some, however rare, that are near to the highest possible realisation of our present humanity. For the march of Nature is not drilled to a regular and mechanical forward stepping. She reaches constantly beyond herself even at the cost of subsequent deplorable retreats. She has rushes; she has splendid and mighty outbursts; she has immense realisations. She storms sometimes passionately forward hoping to take the kingdom of heaven by violence. And these self-exceedings are the revelation of that in her which is most divine or else most diabolical, but in either case the most puissant to bring her rapidly forward towards her goal.

That which Nature has evolved for us and has firmly founded is the bodily life. She has effected a certain combination and harmony of the two inferior but most fundamentally necessary elements of our action and progress upon earth,—Matter, which, however the too ethereally spiritual may despise it, is our foundation and the first condition of all our energies and realisations, and the Life-Energy which is our means of existence in a material body and the basis there even of our mental and spiritual activities. She has successfully achieved a certain stability of her constant material movement which is at once sufficiently steady and durable and sufficiently pliable and mutable to provide a fit dwelling-place and instrument for the progressively manifesting god in humanity. This is what is meant by the fable in the Aitareya Upanishad which tells us that the gods rejected the animal forms successively offered to them by the Divine Self and only when man was produced, cried out, "This indeed is perfectly made," and consented to enter in. She has effected also a working compromise between the inertia of matter and the active Life that lives in and feeds on it, by which not only is vital existence sustained, but the fullest developments of mentality are rendered possible. This equilibrium constitutes the basic status of Nature in man and is termed in the language of Yoga his gross body composed of the material or food sheath and the nervous system or vital vehicle.[1]

If, then, this inferior equilibrium is the basis and first means of the higher movements which the universal Power contemplates and if it constitutes the vehicle in which the Divine here seeks to reveal Itself, if the Indian saying is true that the body is the instrument provided for the fulfilment of the right law of our nature, then any final recoil from the physical life must be a turning away from the completeness of the divine Wisdom and a renunciation of its aim in earthly manifestation. Such a refusal may be, owing to some secret law of their development, the right attitude for certain individuals, but never the aim intended for mankind. It can be, therefore, no integral Yoga which ignores the body or makes its annulment or its rejection indispensable to a perfect spirituality. Rather, the perfecting of the body also should be the last triumph of the Spirit and to make the bodily life also divine must be God's final seal upon His work in the universe. The obstacle which the physical presents to the spiritual is no argument for the rejection of the physical; for in the unseen providence of things our greatest difficulties are our best opportunities. A supreme difficulty is Nature's indication to us of a supreme conquest to be won and an ultimate problem to be solved; it is not a warning of an inextricable snare to be shunned or of an enemy too strong for us from whom we must flee.

Equally, the vital and nervous energies in us are there for a great utility; they too demand the divine realisation of their possibilities in our ultimate fulfilment. The great part assigned to this element in the universal scheme is powerfully emphasised by the catholic wisdom of the Upanishads. "As the spokes of a wheel in its nave, so in the Life-Energy is all established, the triple knowledge and the Sacrifice and the power of the strong and the purity of the wise. Under the control of the LifeEnergy is all this that is established in the triple heaven."[2] It is therefore no integral Yoga that kills these vital energies, forces them into a nerveless quiescence or roots them out as the source of noxious activities. Their purification, not their destruction,—their transformation, control and utilisation is the aim in view with which they have been created and developed in us.

If the bodily life is what Nature has firmly evolved for us as her base and first instrument, it is our mental life that she is evolving as her immediate next aim and superior instrument. This in her ordinary exaltations is the lofty preoccupying thought in her; this, except in her periods of exhaustion and recoil into a reposeful and recuperating obscurity, is her constant pursuit wherever she can get free from the trammels of her first vital and physical realisations. For here in man we have a distinction which is of the utmost importance. He has in him not a single mentality, but a double and a triple, the mind material and nervous, the pure intellectual mind which liberates itself from the illusions of the body and the senses, and a divine mind above intellect which in its turn liberates itself from the imperfect modes of the logically discriminative and imaginative reason. Mind in man is first emmeshed in the life of the body, where in the plant it is entirely involved and in animals always imprisoned. It accepts this life as not only the first but the whole condition of its activities and serves its needs as if they were the entire aim of existence. But the bodily life in man is a base, not the aim, his first condition and not his last determinant. In the just idea of the ancients man is essentially the thinker, the Manu, the mental being who leads the life and the body,[3] not the animal who is led by them. The true human existence, therefore, only begins when the intellectual mentality emerges out of the material and we begin more and more to live in the mind independent of the nervous and physical obsession and in the measure of that liberty are able to accept rightly and rightly to use the life of the body. For freedom and not a skilful subjection is the true means of mastery. A free, not a compulsory acceptance of the conditions, the enlarged and sublimated conditions of our physical being, is the high human ideal. But beyond this intellectual mentality is the divine.

The mental life thus evolving in man is not, indeed, a common possession. In actual appearance it would seem as if it were only developed to the fullest in individuals and as if there were great numbers and even the majority in whom it is either a small and ill-organised part of their normal nature or not evolved at all or latent and not easily made active. Certainly, the mental life is not a finished evolution of Nature; it is not yet firmly founded in the human animal. The sign is that the fine and full equilibrium of vitality and matter, the sane, robust, long-lived human body is ordinarily found only in races or classes of men who reject the effort of thought, its disturbances, its tensions, or think only with the material mind. Civilised man has yet to establish an equilibrium between the fully active mind and the body; he does not normally possess it. Indeed, the increasing effort towards a more intense mental life seems to create, frequently, an increasing disequilibrium of the human elements, so that it is possible for eminent scientists to describe genius as a form of insanity, a result of degeneration, a pathological morbidity of Nature. The phenomena which are used to justify this exaggeration, when taken not separately, but in connection with all other relevant data, point to a different truth. Genius is one attempt of the universal Energy to so quicken and intensify our intellectual powers that they shall be prepared for those more puissant, direct and rapid faculties which constitute the play of the supra-intellectual or divine mind. It is not, then, a freak, an inexplicable phenomenon, but a perfectly natural next step in the right line of her evolution. She has harmonised the bodily life with the material mind, she is harmonising it with the play of the intellectual mentality; for that, although it tends to a depression of the full animal and vital vigour, need not produce active disturbances. And she is shooting yet beyond in the attempt to reach a still higher level. Nor are the disturbances created by her process as great as is often represented. Some of them are the crude beginnings of new manifestations; others are an easily corrected movement of disintegration, often fruitful of fresh activities and always a small price to pay for the far-reaching results that she has in view.

We may perhaps, if we consider all the circumstances, come to this conclusion that mental life, far from being a recent appearance in man, is the swift repetition in him of a previous achievement from which the Energy in the race had undergone one of her deplorable recoils. The savage is perhaps not so much the first forefather of civilised man as the degenerate descendant of a previous civilisation. For if the actuality of intellectual achievement is unevenly distributed, the capacity is spread everywhere. It has been seen that in individual cases even the racial type considered by us the lowest, the negro fresh from the perennial barbarism of Central Africa, is capable, without admixture of blood, without waiting for future generations, of the intellectual culture, if not yet of the intellectual accomplishment of the dominant European. Even in the mass men seem to need, in favourable circumstances, only a few generations to cover ground that ought apparently to be measured in the terms of millenniums. Either, then, man by his privilege as a mental being is exempt from the full burden of the tardy laws of evolution or else he already represents and with helpful conditions and in the right stimulating atmosphere can always display a high level of material capacity for the activities of the intellectual life. It is not mental incapacity, but the long rejection or seclusion from opportunity and withdrawal of the awakening impulse that creates the savage. Barbarism is an intermediate sleep, not an original darkness.

Moreover the whole trend of modern thought and modern endeavour reveals itself to the observant eye as a large conscious effort of Nature in man to effect a general level of intellectual equipment, capacity and farther possibility by universalising the opportunities which modern civilisation affords for the mental life. Even the preoccupation of the European intellect, the protagonist of this tendency, with material Nature and the externalities of existence is a necessary part of the effort. It seeks to prepare a sufficient basis in man's physical being and vital energies and in his material environment for his full mental possibilities. By the spread of education, by the advance of the backward races, by the elevation of depressed classes, by the multiplication of labour-saving appliances, by the movement towards ideal social and economic conditions, by the labour of Science towards an improved health, longevity and sound physique in civilised humanity, the sense and drift of this vast movement translates itself in easily intelligible signs. The right or at least the ultimate means may not always be employed, but their aim is the right preliminary aim,—a sound individual and social body and the satisfaction of the legitimate needs and demands of the material mind, sufficient ease, leisure, equal opportunity, so that the whole of mankind and no longer only the favoured race, class or individual may be free to develop the emotional and intellectual being to its full capacity. At present the material and economic aim may predominate, but always, behind, there works or there waits in reserve the higher and major impulse.

And when the preliminary conditions are satisfied, when the great endeavour has found its base, what will be the nature of that farther possibility which the activities of the intellectual life must serve? If Mind is indeed Nature's highest term, then the entire development of the rational and imaginative intellect and the harmonious satisfaction of the emotions and sensibilities must be to themselves sufficient. But if, on the contrary, man is more than a reasoning and emotional animal, if beyond that which is being evolved, there is something that has to be evolved, then it may well be that the fullness of the mental life, the suppleness, flexibility and wide capacity of the intellect, the ordered richness of emotion and sensibility may be only a passage towards the development of a higher life and of more powerful faculties which are yet to manifest and to take possession of the lower instrument, just as mind itself has so taken possession of the body that the physical being no longer lives only for its own satisfaction but provides the foundation and the materials for a superior activity.

The assertion of a higher than the mental life is the whole foundation of Indian philosophy and its acquisition and organisation is the veritable object served by the methods of Yoga. Mind is not the last term of evolution, not an ultimate aim, but, like body, an instrument. It is even so termed in the language of Yoga, the inner instrument.[4] And Indian tradition asserts that this which is to be manifested is not a new term in human experience, but has been developed before and has even governed humanity in certain periods of its development. In any case, in order to be known it must at one time have been partly developed. And if since then Nature has sunk back from her achievement, the reason must always be found in some unrealised harmony, some insufficiency of the intellectual and material basis to which she has now returned, some over-specialisation of the higher to the detriment of the lower existence.

But what then constitutes this higher or highest existence to which our evolution is tending? In order to answer the question we have to deal with a class of supreme experiences, a class of unusual conceptions which it is difficult to represent accurately in any other language than the ancient Sanskrit tongue in which alone they have been to some extent systematised. The only approximate terms in the English language have other associations and their use may lead to many and even serious inaccuracies. The terminology of Yoga recognises besides the status of our physical and vital being, termed the gross body and doubly composed of the food sheath and the vital vehicle, besides the status of our mental being, termed the subtle body and singly composed of the mind sheath or mental vehicle,[5] a third, supreme and divine status of supra-mental being, termed the causal body and composed of a fourth and a fifth vehicle[6] which are described as those of knowledge and bliss. But this knowledge is not a systematised result of mental questionings and reasonings, not a temporary arrangement of conclusions and opinions in the terms of the highest probability, but rather a pure self-existent and self-luminous Truth. And this bliss is not a supreme pleasure of the heart and sensations with the experience of pain and sorrow as its background, but a delight also self-existent and independent of objects and particular experiences, a self-delight which is the very nature, the very stuff, as it were, of a transcendent and infinite existence.

Do such psychological conceptions correspond to anything real and possible? All Yoga asserts them as its ultimate experience and supreme aim. They form the governing principles of our highest possible state of consciousness, our widest possible range of existence. There is, we say, a harmony of supreme faculties, corresponding roughly to the psychological faculties of revelation, inspiration and intuition, yet acting not in the intuitive reason or the divine mind, but on a still higher plane, which see Truth directly face to face, or rather live in the truth of things both universal and transcendent and are its formulation and luminous activity. And these faculties are the light of a conscious existence superseding the egoistic and itself both cosmic and transcendent, the nature of which is Bliss. These are obviously divine and, as man is at present apparently constituted, superhuman states of consciousness and activity. A trinity of transcendent existence, self-awareness and self-delight[7] is, indeed, the metaphysical description of the supreme Atman, the self-formulation, to our awakened knowledge, of the Unknowable whether conceived as a pure Impersonality or as a cosmic Personality manifesting the universe. But in Yoga they are regarded also in their psychological aspects as states of subjective existence to which our waking consciousness is now alien, but which dwell in us in a superconscious plane and to which, therefore, we may always ascend.

For, as is indicated by the name, causal body (*kāraṇa*), as opposed to the two others which are instruments (*karaṇa*), this crowning manifestation is also the source and effective power of all that in the actual evolution has preceded it. Our mental activities are, indeed, a derivation, selection and, so long as they are divided from the truth that is secretly their source, a deformation of the divine knowledge. Our sensations and emotions have the same relation to the Bliss, our vital forces and actions to the aspect of Will or Force assumed by the divine consciousness, our physical being to the pure essence of that Bliss and Consciousness. The evolution which we observe and of which we are the terrestrial summit may be considered, in a sense, as an inverse manifestation, by which these supreme Powers in their unity and their diversity use, develop and perfect the imperfect substance and activities of Matter, of Life and of Mind so that they, the inferior modes, may express in mutable relativity an increasing harmony of the divine and eternal states from which they are born. If this be the truth of the universe, then the goal of evolution is also its cause, it is that which is immanent in its elements and out of them is liberated. But the liberation is surely imperfect if it is only an escape and there is no return upon the containing substance and activities to exalt and transform them. The immanence itself would have no credible reason for being if it did not end in such a transfiguration. But if human mind can become capable of the glories of the divine Light, human emotion and sensibility can be transformed into the mould and assume the measure and movement of the supreme Bliss, human action not only represent but feel itself to be the motion of a divine and non-egoistic Force and the physical substance of our being sufficiently partake of the purity of the supernal essence, sufficiently unify plasticity and durable constancy to support and prolong these highest experiences and agencies, then all the long labour of Nature will end in a crowning justification and her evolutions reveal their profound significance.

So dazzling is even a glimpse of this supreme existence and so absorbing its attraction that, once seen, we feel readily justified in neglecting all else for its pursuit. Even, by an opposite exaggeration to that which sees all things in Mind and the mental life as an exclusive ideal, Mind comes to be regarded as an unworthy deformation and a supreme obstacle, the source of an illusory universe, a negation of the Truth and itself to be denied and all its works and results annulled if we desire the final liberation. But this is a half-truth which errs by regarding only the actual limitations of Mind and ignores its divine intention. The ultimate knowledge is that which perceives and accepts God in the universe as well as beyond the universe; the integral Yoga is that which, having found the Transcendent, can return upon the universe and possess it, retaining the power freely to descend as well as ascend the great stair of existence. For if the eternal Wisdom exists at all, the faculty of Mind also must have some high use and destiny. That use must depend on its place in the ascent and in the return and that destiny must be a fulfilment and transfiguration, not a rooting out or an annulling.

We perceive, then, these three steps in Nature, a bodily life which is the basis of our existence here in the material world, a mental life into which we emerge and by which we raise the bodily to higher uses and enlarge it into a greater completeness, and a divine existence which is at once the goal of the other two and returns upon them to liberate them into their highest possibilities. Regarding none of them as either beyond our reach or below our nature and the destruction of none of them as essential to the ultimate attainment, we accept this liberation and fulfilment as part at least and a large and important part of the aim of Yoga.

---

1. annakoṣa and prāṇakoṣa.
2. Prasna Upanishad II.
3. manomayaḥ prāṇaśarīranetā. Mundaka Upanishad II. 2. 8.
4. antaḥkaraṇa.
5. manaḥ-koṣa.
6. vijñānakoṣa and ānandakoṣa.
7. saccidānanda.

THE THREEFOLD LIFE

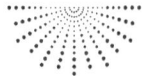

NATURE, then, is an evolution or progressive self-manifestation of an eternal and secret existence, with three successive forms as her three steps of ascent. And we have consequently as the condition of all our activities these three mutually interdependent possibilities, the bodily life, the mental existence and the veiled spiritual being which is in the involution the cause of the others and in the evolution their result. Preserving and perfecting the physical, fulfilling the mental, it is Nature's aim and it should be ours to unveil in the perfected body and mind the transcendent activities of the Spirit. As the mental life does not abrogate but works for the elevation and better utilisation of the bodily existence, so too the spiritual should not abrogate but transfigure our intellectual, emotional, aesthetic and vital activities.

For man, the head of terrestrial Nature, the sole earthly frame in which her full evolution is possible, is a triple birth. He has been given a living frame in which the body is the vessel and life the dynamic means of a divine manifestation. His activity is centred in a progressive mind which aims at perfecting itself as well as the house in which it dwells and the means of life that it uses, and is capable of awaking by a progressive self-realisation to its own true nature as a form of the Spirit. He culminates in what he always really was, the illumined and beatific spirit which is intended at last to irradiate life and mind with its now concealed splendours.

Since this is the plan of the divine Energy in humanity, the whole method and aim of our existence must work by the interaction of these three elements in the being. As a result of their separate formulation in Nature, man has open to him a choice between three kinds of life, the ordinary material existence, a life of mental activity and progress and the unchanging spiritual beatitude. But he can, as he progresses, combine these three forms, resolve their discords into a harmonious rhythm and so create in himself the whole godhead, the perfect Man.

In ordinary Nature they have each their own characteristic and governing impulse.

The characteristic energy of bodily Life is not so much in progress as in persistence, not so much in individual self-enlargement as in self-repetition. There is, indeed, in physical Nature a progression from type to type, from the vegetable to the animal, from the animal to man; for even in inanimate Matter Mind is at work. But once a type is marked off physically, the chief immediate preoccupation of the terrestrial Mother seems to be to keep it in being by a constant reproduction. For Life always seeks immortality; but since individual form is impermanent and only the idea of a form is permanent in the consciousness that creates the universe,—for there it does not perish,—such constant reproduction is the only possible material immortality. Self-preservation, self-repetition, self-multiplication are necessarily, then, the predominant instincts of all material existence. Material life seems ever to move in a fixed cycle.

The characteristic energy of pure Mind is change, and the more our mentality acquires elevation and organisation, the more this law of Mind assumes the aspect of a continual enlargement, improvement and better arrangement of its gains and so of a continual passage from a smaller and simpler to a larger and more complex perfection. For Mind, unlike bodily life, is infinite in its field, elastic in its expansion, easily variable in its formations. Change, then, self-enlargement and self-improvement are its proper instincts. Mind too moves in cycles, but these are ever-enlarging spirals. Its faith is perfectibility, its watchword is progress.

The characteristic law of Spirit is self-existent perfection and immutable infinity. It possesses always and in its own right the immortality which is the aim of Life and the perfection which is the goal of Mind. The attainment of the eternal and the realisation of that which is the same in all things and beyond all things, equally blissful in universe and outside it, untouched by the imperfections and limitations of the forms and activities in which it dwells, are the glory of the spiritual life.

In each of these forms Nature acts both individually and collectively; for the Eternal affirms Himself equally in the single form and in the group-existence, whether family, clan and nation or groupings dependent on less physical principles or the supreme group of all, our collective humanity. Man also may seek his own individual good from any or all of these spheres of activity, or identify himself in them with the collectivity and live for it, or, rising to a truer perception of this complex universe, harmonise the individual realisation with the collective aim. For as it is the right relation of the soul with the Supreme, while it is in the universe, neither to assert egoistically its separate being nor to blot itself out in the Indefinable, but to realise its unity with the Divine and the world and unite them in the individual, so the right relation of the individual with the collectivity is neither to pursue egoistically his own material or mental progress or spiritual salvation without regard to his fellows, nor for the sake of the community to suppress or maim his proper development, but to sum up in himself all its best and completest possibilities and pour them out by thought, action and all other means on his surroundings so that the whole race may approach nearer to the attainment of its supreme personalities.

It follows that the object of the material life must be to fulfil, above all things, the vital aim of Nature. The whole aim of the material man is to live, to pass from birth to death with as much comfort or enjoyment as may be on the way, but anyhow to live. He can subordinate this aim, but only to physical Nature's other instincts, the reproduction of the individual and the conservation of the type in the family, class or community. Self, domesticity, the accustomed order of the society and of the nation are the constituents of the material existence. Its immense importance in the economy of Nature is self-evident, and commensurate is the importance of the human type which represents it. He assures her of the safety of the framework she has made and of the orderly continuance and conservation of her past gains.

But by that very utility such men and the life they lead are condemned to be limited, irrationally conservative and earthbound. The customary routine, the customary institutions, the inherited or habitual forms of thought,—these things are the life-breath of their nostrils. They admit and jealously defend the changes compelled by the progressive mind in the past, but combat with equal zeal the changes that are being made by it in the present. For to the material man the living progressive thinker is an ideologue, dreamer or madman. The old Semites who stoned the living prophets and adored their memories when dead, were the very incarnation of this instinctive and unintelligent principle in Nature. In the ancient Indian distinction between the once born and the twice born, it is to this material man that the former description can be applied. He does Nature's inferior works; he assures the basis for her higher activities; but not to him easily are opened the glories of her second birth.

Yet he admits so much of spirituality as has been enforced on his customary ideas by the great religious outbursts of the past and he makes in his scheme of society a place, venerable though not often effective, for the priest or the learned theologian who can be trusted to provide him with a safe and ordinary spiritual pabulum. But to the man who would assert for himself the liberty of spiritual experience and the spiritual life, he assigns, if he admits him at all, not the vestment of the priest but the robe of the Sannyasin. Outside society let him exercise his dangerous freedom. So he may even serve as a human lightning-rod receiving the electricity of the Spirit and turning it away from the social edifice.

Nevertheless it is possible to make the material man and his life moderately progressive by imprinting on the material mind the custom of progress, the habit of conscious change, the fixed idea of progression as a law of life. The creation by this means of progressive societies in Europe is one of the greatest triumphs of Mind over Matter. But the physical nature has its revenge; for the progress made tends to be of the grosser and more outward kind and its attempts at a higher or a more rapid movement bring about great wearinesses, swift exhaustions, startling recoils.

It is possible also to give the material man and his life a moderate spirituality by accustoming him to regard in a religious spirit all the institutions of life and its customary activities. The creation of such spiritualised communities in the East has been one of the greatest triumphs of Spirit over Matter. Yet here, too, there is a defect; for this often tends only to the creation of a religious temperament, the most outward form of spirituality. Its higher manifestations, even the most splendid and puissant, either merely increase the number of souls drawn out of social life and so impoverish it or disturb the society for a while by a momentary elevation. The truth is that neither the mental effort nor the spiritual impulse can suffice, divorced from each other, to overcome the immense resistance of material Nature. She demands their alliance in a complete effort before she will suffer a complete change in humanity. But, usually, these two great agents are unwilling to make to each other the necessary concessions.

The mental life concentrates on the aesthetic, the ethical and the intellectual activities. Essential mentality is idealistic and a seeker after perfection. The subtle self, the brilliant Atman,[1] is ever a dreamer. A dream of perfect beauty, perfect conduct, perfect Truth, whether seeking new forms of the Eternal or revitalising the old, is the very soul of pure mentality. But it knows not how to deal with the resistance of Matter. There it is hampered and inefficient, works by bungling experiments and has either to withdraw from the struggle or submit to the grey actuality. Or else, by studying the material life and accepting the conditions of the contest, it may succeed, but only in imposing temporarily some artificial system which infinite Nature either rends and casts aside or disfigures out of recognition or by withdrawing her assent leaves as the corpse of a dead ideal. Few and far between have been those realisations of the dreamer in Man which the world has gladly accepted, looks back to with a fond memory and seeks, in its elements, to cherish.

When the gulf between actual life and the temperament of the thinker is too great, we see as the result a sort of withdrawing of the Mind from life in order to act with a greater freedom in its own sphere. The poet living among his brilliant visions, the artist absorbed in his art, the philosopher thinking out the problems of the intellect in his solitary chamber, the scientist, the scholar caring only for their studies and their experiments, were often in former days, are even now not unoften the Sannyasins of the intellect. To the work they have done for humanity, all its past bears record.

But such seclusion is justified only by some special activity. Mind finds fully its force and action only when it casts itself upon life and accepts equally its possibilities and its resistances as the means of a greater self-perfection. In the struggle with the difficulties of the material world the ethical development of the individual is firmly shaped and the great schools of conduct are formed; by contact with the facts of life Art attains to vitality, Thought assures its abstractions, the generalisations of the philosopher base themselves on a stable foundation of science and experience.

This mixing with life may, however, be pursued for the sake of the individual mind and with an entire indifference to the forms of the material existence or the uplifting of the race. This indifference is seen at its highest in the Epicurean discipline and is not entirely absent from the Stoic; and even altruism does the works of compassion more often for its own sake than for the sake of the world it helps. But this too is a limited fulfilment. The progressive mind is seen at its noblest when it strives to elevate the whole race to its own level whether by sowing broadcast the image of its own thought and fulfilment or by changing the material life of the race into fresh forms, religious, intellectual, social or political, intended to represent more nearly that ideal of truth, beauty, justice, righteousness with which the man's own soul is illumined. Failure in such a field matters little; for the mere attempt is dynamic and creative. The struggle of Mind to elevate life is the promise and condition of the conquest of life by that which is higher even than Mind.

That highest thing, the spiritual existence, is concerned with what is eternal but not therefore entirely aloof from the transient. For the spiritual man the mind's dream of perfect beauty is realised in an eternal love, beauty and delight that has no dependence and is equal behind all objective appearances; its dream of perfect Truth in the supreme, self-existent, self-apparent and eternal Verity which never varies, but explains and is the secret of all variations and the goal of all progress; its dream of perfect action in the omnipotent and self-guiding Law that is inherent for ever in all things and translates itself here in the rhythm of the worlds. What is fugitive vision or constant effort of creation in the brilliant Self is an eternally existing Reality in the Self that knows[2] and is the Lord.

But if it is often difficult for the mental life to accommodate itself to the dully resistant material activity, how much more difficult must it seem for the spiritual existence to live on in a world that appears full not of the Truth but of every lie and illusion, not of Love and Beauty but of an encompassing discord and ugliness, not of the Law of Truth but of victorious selfishness and sin? Therefore the spiritual life tends easily in the saint and Sannyasin to withdraw from the material existence and reject it either wholly and physically or in the spirit. It sees this world as the kingdom of evil or of ignorance and the eternal and divine either in a far-off heaven or beyond where there is no world and no life. It separates itself inwardly, if not also physically, from the world's impurities; it asserts the spiritual reality in a spotless isolation. This withdrawal renders an invaluable service to the material life itself by forcing it to regard and even to bow down to something that is the direct negation of its own petty ideals, sordid cares and egoistic self-content.

But the work in the world of so supreme a power as spiritual force cannot be thus limited. The spiritual life also can return upon the material and use it as a means of its own greater fullness. Refusing to be blinded by the dualities, the appearances, it can seek in all appearances whatsoever the vision of the same Lord, the same eternal Truth, Beauty, Love, Delight. The Vedantic formula of the Self in all things, all things in the Self and all things as becomings of the Self is the key to this richer and all-embracing Yoga.

But the spiritual life, like the mental, may thus make use of this outward existence for the benefit of the individual with a perfect indifference to any collective uplifting of the merely symbolic world which it uses. Since the Eternal is for ever the same in all things and all things the same to the Eternal, since the exact mode of action and the result are of no importance compared with the working out in oneself of the one great realisation, this spiritual indifference accepts no matter what environment, no matter what action, dispassionately, prepared to retire as soon as its own supreme end is realised. It is so that many have understood the ideal of the Gita. Or else the inner love and bliss may pour itself out on the world in good deeds, in service, in compassion, the inner Truth in the giving of knowledge, without therefore attempting the transformation of a world which must by its inalienable nature remain a battlefield of the dualities, of sin and virtue, of truth and error, of joy and suffering.

But if Progress also is one of the chief terms of world-existence and a progressive manifestation of the Divine the true sense of Nature, this limitation also is invalid. It is possible for the spiritual life in the world, and it is its real mission, to change the material life into its own image, the image of the Divine. Therefore, besides the great solitaries who have sought and attained their self-liberation, we have the great spiritual teachers who have also liberated others and, supreme of all, the great dynamic souls who, feeling themselves stronger in the might of the Spirit than all the forces of the material life banded together, have thrown themselves upon the world, grappled with it in a loving wrestle and striven to compel its consent to its own transfiguration. Ordinarily, the effort is concentrated on a mental and moral change in humanity, but it may extend itself also to the alteration of the forms of our life and its institutions so that they too may be a better mould for the inpourings of the Spirit. These attempts have been the supreme landmarks in the progressive development of human ideals and the divine preparation of the race. Every one of them, whatever its outward results, has left Earth more capable of Heaven and quickened in its tardy movements the evolutionary Yoga of Nature.

In India, for the last thousand years and more, the spiritual life and the material have existed side by side to the exclusion of the progressive mind. Spirituality has made terms for itself with Matter by renouncing the attempt at general progress. It has obtained from society the right of free spiritual development for all who assume some distinctive symbol, such as the garb of the Sannyasin, the recognition of that life as man's goal and those who live it as worthy of an absolute reverence, and the casting of society itself into such a religious mould that its most customary acts should be accompanied by a formal reminder of the spiritual symbolism of life and its ultimate destination. On the other hand, there was conceded to society the right of inertia and immobile self-conservation. The concession destroyed much of the value of the terms. The religious mould being fixed, the formal reminder tended to become a routine and to lose its living sense. The constant attempts to change the mould by new sects and religions ended only in a new routine or a modification of the old; for the saving element of the free and active mind had been exiled. The material life, handed over to the Ignorance, the purposeless and endless duality, became a leaden and dolorous yoke from which flight was the only escape.

The schools of Indian Yoga lent themselves to the compromise. Individual perfection or liberation was made the aim, seclusion of some kind from the ordinary activities the condition, the renunciation of life the culmination. The teacher gave his knowledge only to a small circle of disciples. Or if a wider movement was attempted, it was still the release of the individual soul that remained the aim. The pact with an immobile society was, for the most part, observed.

The utility of the compromise in the then actual state of the world cannot be doubted. It secured in India a society which lent itself to the preservation and the worship of spirituality, a country apart in which as in a fortress the highest spiritual ideal could maintain itself in its most absolute purity unoverpowered by the siege of the forces around it. But it was a compromise, not an absolute victory. The material life lost the divine impulse to growth, the spiritual preserved by isolation its height and purity, but sacrificed its full power and serviceableness to the world. Therefore, in the divine Providence the country of the Yogins and the Sannyasins has been forced into a strict and imperative contact with the very element it had rejected, the element of the progressive Mind, so that it might recover what was now wanting to it.

We have to recognise once more that the individual exists not in himself alone but in the collectivity and that individual perfection and liberation are not the whole sense of God's intention in the world. The free use of our liberty includes also the liberation of others and of mankind; the perfect utility of our perfection is, having realised in ourselves the divine symbol, to reproduce, multiply and ultimately universalise it in others.

Therefore from a concrete view of human life in its threefold potentialities we come to the same conclusion that we had drawn from an observation of Nature in her general workings and the three steps of her evolution. And we begin to perceive a complete aim for our synthesis of Yoga.

Spirit is the crown of universal existence; Matter is its basis; Mind is the link between the two. Spirit is that which is eternal; Mind and Matter are its workings. Spirit is that which is concealed and has to be revealed; mind and body are the means by which it seeks to reveal itself. Spirit is the image of the Lord of the Yoga; mind and body are the means He has provided for reproducing that image in phenomenal existence. All Nature is an attempt at a progressive revelation of the concealed Truth, a more and more successful reproduction of the divine image.

But what Nature aims at for the mass in a slow evolution, Yoga effects for the individual by a rapid revolution. It works by a quickening of all her energies, a sublimation of all her faculties. While she develops the spiritual life with difficulty and has constantly to fall back from it for the sake of her lower realisations, the sublimated force, the concentrated method of Yoga can attain directly and carry with it the perfection of the mind and even, if she will, the perfection of the body. Nature seeks the Divine in her own symbols: Yoga goes beyond Nature to the Lord of Nature, beyond universe to the Transcendent and can return with the transcendent light and power, with the fiat of the Omnipotent.

But their aim is one in the end. The generalisation of Yoga in humanity must be the last victory of Nature over her own delays and concealments. Even as now by the progressive mind in Science she seeks to make all mankind fit for the full development of the mental life, so by Yoga must she inevitably seek to make all mankind fit for the higher evolution, the second birth, the spiritual existence. And as the mental life uses and perfects the material, so will the spiritual use and perfect the material and the mental existence as the instruments of a divine self-expression. The ages when that is accomplished, are the legendary Satya or Krita[3] Yugas, the ages of the Truth manifested in the symbol, of the great work done when Nature in mankind, illumined, satisfied and blissful, rests in the culmination of her endeavour.

It is for man to know her meaning, no longer misunderstanding, vilifying or misusing the universal Mother, and to aspire always by her mightiest means to her highest ideal.

1. Who dwells in Dream, the inly conscious, the enjoyer of abstractions, the Brilliant. Mandukya Upanishad 4.
2. The Unified, in whom conscious thought is concentrated, who is all delight and enjoyer of delight, the Wise. . . . He is the Lord of all, the Omniscient, the inner Guide. Mandukya Upanishad 5, 6.
3. Satya means Truth; Krita, effected or completed.

THE SYSTEMS OF YOGA

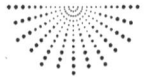

THESE relations between the different psychological divisions of the human being and these various utilities and objects of effort founded on them, such as we have seen them in our brief survey of the natural evolution, we shall find repeated in the fundamental principles and methods of the different schools of Yoga. And if we seek to combine and harmonise their central practices and their predominant aims, we shall find that the basis provided by Nature is still our natural basis and the condition of their synthesis.

In one respect Yoga exceeds the normal operation of cosmic Nature and climbs beyond her. For the aim of the Universal Mother is to embrace the Divine in her own play and creations and there to realise It. But in the highest flights of Yoga she reaches beyond herself and realises the Divine in Itself exceeding the universe and even standing apart from the cosmic play. Therefore by some it is supposed that this is not only the highest but also the one true or exclusively preferable object of Yoga.

Yet it is always through something which she has formed in her evolution that Nature thus overpasses her evolution. It is the individual heart that by sublimating its highest and purest emotions attains to the transcendent Bliss or the ineffable Nirvana, the individual mind that by converting its ordinary functionings into a knowledge beyond mentality knows its oneness with the Ineffable and merges its separate existence in that transcendent unity. And always it is the individual, the Self conditioned in its experience by Nature and working through her formations, that attains to the Self unconditioned, free and transcendent.

In practice three conceptions are necessary before there can be any possibility of Yoga; there must be, as it were, three consenting parties to the effort,—God, Nature and the human soul or, in more abstract language, the Transcendental, the Universal and the Individual. If the individual and Nature are left to themselves, the one is bound to the other and unable to exceed appreciably her lingering march. Something transcendent is needed, free from her and greater, which will act upon us and her, attracting us upward to Itself and securing from her by good grace or by force her consent to the individual ascension.

It is this truth which makes necessary to every philosophy of Yoga the conception of the Ishwara, Lord, supreme Soul or supreme Self, towards whom the effort is directed and who gives the illuminating touch and the strength to attain. Equally true is the complementary idea so often enforced by the Yoga of devotion that as the Transcendent is necessary to the individual and sought after by him, so also the individual is necessary in a sense to the Transcendent and sought after by It. If the Bhakta seeks and yearns after Bhagavan, Bhagavan also seeks and yearns after the Bhakta.[1] There can be no Yoga of knowledge without a human seeker of the knowledge, the supreme subject of knowledge and the divine use by the individual of the universal faculties of knowledge; no Yoga of devotion without the human God-lover, the supreme object of love and delight and the divine use by the individual of the universal faculties of spiritual, emotional and aesthetic enjoyment; no Yoga of works without the human worker, the supreme Will, Master of all works and sacrifices, and the divine use by the individual of the universal faculties of power and action. However Monistic may be our intellectual conception of the highest truth of things, in practice we are compelled to accept this omnipresent Trinity.

For the contact of the human and individual consciousness with the divine is the very essence of Yoga. Yoga is the union of that which has become separated in the play of the universe with its own true self, origin and universality. The contact may take place at any point of the complex and intricately organised consciousness which we call our personality. It may be effected in the physical through the body; in the vital through the action of those functionings which determine the state and the experiences of our nervous being; through the mentality, whether by means of the emotional heart, the active will or the understanding mind, or more largely by a general conversion of the mental consciousness in all its activities. It may equally be accomplished through a direct awakening to the universal or transcendent Truth and Bliss by the conversion of the central ego in the mind. And according to the point of contact that we choose will be the type of the Yoga that we practise.

For if, leaving aside the complexities of their particular processes, we fix our regard on the central principle of the chief schools of Yoga still prevalent in India, we find that they arrange themselves in an ascending order which starts from the lowest rung of the ladder, the body, and ascends to the direct contact between the individual soul and the transcendent and universal Self. Hathayoga selects the body and the vital functionings as its instruments of perfection and realisation; its concern is with the gross body. Rajayoga selects the mental being in its different parts as its lever-power; it concentrates on the subtle body. The triple Path of Works, of Love and of Knowledge uses some part of the mental being, will, heart or intellect as a starting-point and seeks by its conversion to arrive at the liberating Truth, Beatitude and Infinity which are the nature of the spiritual life. Its method is a direct commerce between the human Purusha in the individual body and the divine Purusha who dwells in every body and yet transcends all form and name.

Hathayoga aims at the conquest of the life and the body whose combination in the food sheath and the vital vehicle constitutes, as we have seen, the gross body and whose equilibrium is the foundation of all Nature's workings in the human being. The equilibrium established by Nature is sufficient for the normal egoistic life; it is insufficient for the purpose of the Hathayogin. For it is calculated on the amount of vital or dynamic force necessary to drive the physical engine during the normal span of human life and to perform more or less adequately the various workings demanded of it by the individual life inhabiting this frame and the world-environment by which it is conditioned.

Hathayoga therefore seeks to rectify Nature and establish another equilibrium by which the physical frame will be able to sustain the inrush of an increasing vital or dynamic force of Prana indefinite, almost infinite in its quantity or intensity. In Nature the equilibrium is based upon the individualisation of a limited quantity and force of the Prana; more than that the individual is by personal and hereditary habit unable to bear, use or control. In Hathayoga, the equilibrium opens a door to the universalisation of the individual vitality by admitting into the body, containing, using and controlling a much less fixed and limited action of the universal energy.

The chief processes of Hathayoga are *āsana* and *prāṇāyāma*. By its numerous *āsanas* or fixed postures it first cures the body of that restlessness which is a sign of its inability to contain without working them off in action and movement the vital forces poured into it from the universal Life-Ocean, gives to it an extraordinary health, force and suppleness and seeks to liberate it from the habits by which it is subjected to ordinary physical Nature and kept within the narrow bounds of her normal operations. In the ancient tradition of Hathayoga it has always been supposed that this conquest could be pushed so far even as to conquer to a great extent the force of gravitation. By various subsidiary but elaborate processes the Hathayogin next contrives to keep the body free from all impurities and the nervous system unclogged for those exercises of respiration which are his most important instruments. These are called *prāṇāyāma*, the control of the breath or vital power; for breathing is the chief physical functioning of the vital forces. Pranayama, for the Hathayogin, serves a double purpose. First, it completes the perfection of the body. The vitality is liberated from many of the ordinary necessities of physical Nature; robust health, prolonged youth, often an extraordinary longevity are attained. On the other hand, Pranayama awakens the coiled-up serpent of the Pranic dynamism in the vital sheath and opens to the Yogin fields of consciousness, ranges of experience, abnormal faculties denied to the ordinary human life while it puissantly intensifies such normal powers and faculties as he already possesses.

These advantages can be farther secured and emphasised by other subsidiary processes open to the Hathayogin.

The results of Hathayoga are thus striking to the eye and impose easily on the vulgar or physical mind. And yet at the end we may ask what we have gained at the end of all this stupendous labour. The object of physical Nature, the preservation of the mere physical life, its highest perfection, even in a certain sense the capacity of a greater enjoyment of physical living have been carried out on an abnormal scale. But the weakness of Hathayoga is that its laborious and difficult processes make so great a demand on the time and energy and impose so complete a severance from the ordinary life of men that the utilisation of its results for the life of the world becomes either impracticable or is extraordinarily restricted. If in return for this loss we gain another life in another world within, the mental, the dynamic, these results could have been acquired through other systems, through Rajayoga, through Tantra, by much less laborious methods and held on much less exacting terms. On the other hand the physical results, increased vitality, prolonged youth, health, longevity are of small avail if they must be held by us as misers of ourselves, apart from the common life, for their own sake, not utilised, not thrown into the common sum of the world's activities. Hathayoga attains large results, but at an exorbitant price and to very little purpose.

Rajayoga takes a higher flight. It aims at the liberation and perfection not of the bodily, but of the mental being, the control of the emotional and sensational life, the mastery of the whole apparatus of thought and consciousness. It fixes its eyes on the *citta*, that stuff of mental consciousness in which all these activities arise, and it seeks, even as Hathayoga with its physical material, first to purify and to tranquillise. The normal state of man is a condition of trouble and disorder, a kingdom either at war with itself or badly governed; for the lord, the Purusha, is subjected to his ministers, the faculties, subjected even to his subjects, the instruments of sensation, emotion, action, enjoyment. Swarajya, self-rule, must be substituted for this subjection. First, therefore, the powers of order must be helped to overcome the powers of disorder. The preliminary movement of Rajayoga is a careful self-discipline by which good habits of mind are substituted for the lawless movements that indulge the lower nervous being. By the practice of truth, by renunciation of all forms of egoistic seeking, by abstention from injury to others, by purity, by constant meditation and inclination to the divine Purusha who is the true lord of the mental kingdom, a pure, glad, clear state of mind and heart is established.

This is the first step only. Afterwards, the ordinary activities of the mind and sense must be entirely quieted in order that the soul may be free to ascend to higher states of consciousness and acquire the foundation for a perfect freedom and self-mastery. But Rajayoga does not forget that the disabilities of the ordinary mind proceed largely from its subjection to the reactions of the nervous system and the body. It adopts therefore from the Hathayogic system its devices of *āsana* and *prāṇāyāma*, but reduces their multiple and elaborate forms in each case to one simplest and most directly effective process sufficient for its own immediate object. Thus it gets rid of the Hathayogic complexity and cumbrousness while it utilises the swift and powerful efficacy of its methods for the control of the body and the vital functions and for the awakening of that internal dynamism, full of a latent supernormal faculty, typified in Yogic terminology by the *kuṇḍalinī*, the coiled and sleeping serpent of Energy within. This done, the system proceeds to the perfect quieting of the restless mind and its elevation to a higher plane through concentration of mental force by the successive stages which lead to the utmost inner concentration or ingathered state of the consciousness which is called Samadhi.

By Samadhi, in which the mind acquires the capacity of withdrawing from its limited waking activities into freer and higher states of consciousness, Rajayoga serves a double purpose. It compasses a pure mental action liberated from the confusions of the outer consciousness and passes thence to the higher supra-mental planes on which the individual soul enters into its true spiritual existence. But also it acquires the capacity of that free and concentrated energising of consciousness on its object which our philosophy asserts as the primary cosmic energy and the method of divine action upon the world. By this capacity the Yogin, already possessed of the highest supracosmic knowledge and experience in the state of trance, is able in the waking state to acquire directly whatever knowledge and exercise whatever mastery may be useful or necessary to his activities in the objective world. For the ancient system of Rajayoga aimed not only at Swarajya, self-rule or subjective empire, the entire control by the subjective consciousness of all the states and activities proper to its own domain, but included Samrajya as well, outward empire, the control by the subjective consciousness of its outer activities and environment.

We perceive that as Hathayoga, dealing with the life and body, aims at the supernormal perfection of the physical life and its capacities and goes beyond it into the domain of the mental life, so Rajayoga, operating with the mind, aims at a supernormal perfection and enlargement of the capacities of the mental life and goes beyond it into the domain of the spiritual existence. But the weakness of the system lies in its excessive reliance on abnormal states of trance. This limitation leads first to a certain aloofness from the physical life which is our foundation and the sphere into which we have to bring our mental and spiritual gains. Especially is the spiritual life, in this system, too much associated with the state of Samadhi. Our object is to make the spiritual life and its experiences fully active and fully utilisable in the waking state and even in the normal use of the functions. But in Rajayoga it tends to withdraw into a subliminal plane at the back of our normal experiences instead of descending and possessing our whole existence.

The triple Path of devotion, knowledge and works attempts the province which Rajayoga leaves unoccupied. It differs from Rajayoga in that it does not occupy itself with the elaborate training of the whole mental system as the condition of perfection, but seizes on certain central principles, the intellect, the heart, the will, and seeks to convert their normal operations by turning them away from their ordinary and external preoccupation and activities and concentrating them on the Divine. It differs also in this,—and here from the point of view of an integral Yoga there seems to be a defect,—that it is indifferent to mental and bodily perfection and aims only at purity as a condition of the divine realisation. A second defect is that as actually practised it chooses one of the three parallel paths exclusively and almost in antagonism to the others instead of effecting a synthetic harmony of the intellect, the heart and the will in an integral divine realisation.

The Path of Knowledge aims at the realisation of the unique and supreme Self. It proceeds by the method of intellectual reflection, *vicāra*, to right discrimination, *viveka*. It observes and distinguishes the different elements of our apparent or phenomenal being and rejecting identification with each of them arrives at their exclusion and separation in one common term as constituents of Prakriti, of phenomenal Nature, creations of Maya, the phenomenal consciousness. So it is able to arrive at its right identification with the pure and unique Self which is not mutable or perishable, not determinable by any phenomenon or combination of phenomena. From this point the path, as ordinarily followed, leads to the rejection of the phenomenal worlds from the consciousness as an illusion and the final immergence without return of the individual soul in the Supreme.

But this exclusive consummation is not the sole or inevitable result of the Path of Knowledge. For, followed more largely and with a less individual aim, the method of Knowledge may lead to an active conquest of the cosmic existence for the Divine no less than to a transcendence. The point of this departure is the realisation of the supreme Self not only in one's own being but in all beings and, finally, the realisation of even the phenomenal aspects of the world as a play of the divine consciousness and not something entirely alien to its true nature. And on the basis of this realisation a yet further enlargement is possible, the conversion of all forms of knowledge, however mundane, into activities of the divine consciousness utilisable for the perception of the one and unique Object of knowledge both in itself and through the play of its forms and symbols. Such a method might well lead to the elevation of the whole range of human intellect and perception to the divine level, to its spiritualisation and to the justification of the cosmic travail of knowledge in humanity. The Path of Devotion aims at the enjoyment of the supreme Love and Bliss and utilises normally the conception of the supreme Lord in His personality as the divine Lover and enjoyer of the universe. The world is then realised as a play of the Lord, with our human life as its final stage, pursued through the different phases of self-concealment and self-revelation. The principle of Bhakti Yoga is to utilise all the normal relations of human life into which emotion enters and apply them no longer to transient worldly relations, but to the joy of the All-Loving, the All-Beautiful and the All-Blissful. Worship and meditation are used only for the preparation and increase of intensity of the divine relationship. And this Yoga is catholic in its use of all emotional relations, so that even enmity and opposition to God, considered as an intense, impatient and perverse form of Love, is conceived as a possible means of realisation and salvation. This path, too, as ordinarily practised, leads away from world-existence to an absorption, of another kind than the Monist's, in the Transcendent and Supra-cosmic.

But, here too, the exclusive result is not inevitable. The Yoga itself provides a first corrective by not confining the play of divine love to the relation between the supreme Soul and the individual, but extending it to a common feeling and mutual worship between the devotees themselves united in the same realisation of the supreme Love and Bliss. It provides a yet more general corrective in the realisation of the divine object of Love in all beings not only human but animal, easily extended to all forms whatsoever. We can see how this larger application of the Yoga of Devotion may be so used as to lead to the elevation of the whole range of human emotion, sensation and aesthetic perception to the divine level, its spiritualisation and the justification of the cosmic labour towards love and joy in our humanity.

The Path of Works aims at the dedication of every human activity to the supreme Will. It begins by the renunciation of all egoistic aim for our works, all pursuit of action for an interested aim or for the sake of a worldly result. By this renunciation it so purifies the mind and the will that we become easily conscious of the great universal Energy as the true doer of all our actions and the Lord of that Energy as their ruler and director with the individual as only a mask, an excuse, an instrument or, more positively, a conscious centre of action and phenomenal relation. The choice and direction of the act is more and more consciously left to this supreme Will and this universal Energy. To That our works as well as the results of our works are finally abandoned. The object is the release of the soul from its bondage to appearances and to the reaction of phenomenal activities. Karmayoga is used, like the other paths, to lead to liberation from phenomenal existence and a departure into the Supreme. But here too the exclusive result is not inevitable. The end of the path may be, equally, a perception of the Divine in all energies, in all happenings, in all activities, and a free and unegoistic participation of the soul in the cosmic action. So followed it will lead to the elevation of all human will and activity to the divine level, its spiritualisation and the justification of the cosmic labour towards freedom, power and perfection in the human being.

We can see also that in the integral view of things these three paths are one. Divine Love should normally lead to the perfect knowledge of the Beloved by perfect intimacy, thus becoming a path of Knowledge, and to divine service, thus becoming a path of Works. So also should perfect Knowledge lead to perfect Love and Joy and a full acceptance of the works of That which is known; dedicated Works to the entire love of the Master of the Sacrifice and the deepest knowledge of His ways and His being. It is in this triple path that we come most readily to the absolute knowledge, love and service of the One in all beings and in the entire cosmic manifestation.

---

1. Bhakta, the devotee or lover of God; Bhagavan, God, the Lord of Love and Delight. The third term of the trinity is Bhagavat, the divine revelation of Love.

THE SYNTHESIS OF THE SYSTEMS

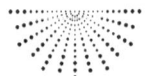

BY THE very nature of the principal Yogic schools, each covering in its operations a part of the complex human integer and attempting to bring out its highest possibilities, it will appear that a synthesis of all of them largely conceived and applied might well result in an integral Yoga. But they are so disparate in their tendencies, so highly specialised and elaborated in their forms, so long confirmed in the mutual opposition of their ideas and methods that we do not easily find how we can arrive at their right union.

    An undiscriminating combination in block would not be a synthesis, but a confusion. Nor would a successive practice of each of them in turn be easy in the short span of our human life and with our limited energies, to say nothing of the waste of labour implied in so cumbrous a process. Sometimes, indeed, Hathayoga and Rajayoga are thus successively practised. And in a recent unique example, in the life of Ramakrishna Paramhansa, we see a colossal spiritual capacity first driving straight to the divine realisation, taking, as it were, the kingdom of heaven by violence, and then seizing upon one Yogic method after another and extracting the substance out of it with an incredible rapidity, always to return to the heart of the whole matter, the realisation and possession of God by the power of love, by the extension of inborn spirituality into various experience and by the spontaneous play of an intuitive knowledge. Such an example cannot be generalised. Its object also was special and temporal, to exemplify in the great and decisive experience of a master-soul the truth, now most necessary to humanity, towards which a world long divided into jarring sects and schools is with difficulty labouring, that all sects are forms and fragments of a single integral truth and all disciplines labour in their different ways towards one supreme experience. To know, be and possess the Divine is the one thing needful and it includes or leads up to all the rest; towards this sole good we have to drive and this attained, all the rest that the divine Will chooses for us, all necessary form and manifestation, will be added.

The synthesis we propose cannot, then, be arrived at either by combination in mass or by successive practice. It must therefore be effected by neglecting the forms and outsides of the Yogic disciplines and seizing rather on some central principle common to all which will include and utilise in the right place and proportion their particular principles, and on some central dynamic force which is the common secret of their divergent methods and capable therefore of organising a natural selection and combination of their varied energies and different utilities. This was the aim which we set before ourselves at first when we entered upon our comparative examination of the methods of Nature and the methods of Yoga and we now return to it with the possibility of hazarding some definite solution.

We observe, first, that there still exists in India a remarkable Yogic system which is in its nature synthetical and starts from a great central principle of Nature, a great dynamic force of Nature; but it is a Yoga apart, not a synthesis of other schools. This system is the way of the Tantra. Owing to certain of its developments Tantra has fallen into discredit with those who are not Tantrics; and especially owing to the developments of its left-hand path, the Vama Marga, which not content with exceeding the duality of virtue and sin and instead of replacing them by spontaneous rightness of action seemed, sometimes, to make a method of self-indulgence, a method of unrestrained social immorality. Nevertheless, in its origin, Tantra was a great and puissant system founded upon ideas which were at least partially true. Even its twofold division into the right-hand and left-hand paths, Dakshina Marga and Vama Marga, started from a certain profound perception. In the ancient symbolic sense of the words Dakshina and Vama, it was the distinction between the way of Knowledge and the way of Ananda,—Nature in man liberating itself by right discrimination in power and practice of its own energies, elements and potentialities and Nature in man liberating itself by joyous acceptance in power and practice of its own energies, elements and potentialities. But in both paths there was in the end an obscuration of principles, a deformation of symbols and a fall.

If, however, we leave aside, here also, the actual methods and practices and seek for the central principle, we find, first, that Tantra expressly differentiates itself from the Vedic methods of Yoga. In a sense, all the schools we have hitherto examined are Vedantic in their principle; their force is in knowledge, their method is knowledge, though it is not always discernment by the intellect, but may be, instead, the knowledge of the heart expressed in love and faith or a knowledge in the will working out through action. In all of them the lord of the Yoga is the Purusha, the Conscious Soul that knows, observes, attracts, governs. But in Tantra it is rather Prakriti, the Nature-Soul, the Energy, the Will-in-Power executive in the universe. It was by learning and applying the intimate secrets of this Will-in-Power, its method, its Tantra, that the Tantric Yogin pursued the aims of his discipline,—mastery, perfection, liberation, beatitude. Instead of drawing back from manifested Nature and its difficulties, he confronted them, seized and conquered. But in the end, as is the general tendency of Prakriti, Tantric Yoga largely lost its principle in its machinery and became a thing of formulae and occult mechanism still powerful when rightly used but fallen from the clarity of their original intention.

We have in this central Tantric conception one side of the truth, the worship of the Energy, the Shakti, as the sole effective force for all attainment. We get the other extreme in the Vedantic conception of the Shakti as a power of Illusion and in the search after the silent inactive Purusha as the means of liberation from the deceptions created by the active Energy. But in the integral conception the Conscious Soul is the Lord, the Nature-Soul is his executive Energy. Purusha is of the nature of Sat, the being of conscious self-existence pure and infinite; Shakti or Prakriti is of the nature of Chit,—it is power of the Purusha's self-conscious existence, pure and infinite. The relation of the two exists between the poles of rest and action. When the Energy is absorbed in the bliss of conscious self-existence, there is rest; when the Purusha pours itself out in the action of its Energy, there is action, creation and the enjoyment or Ananda of becoming. But if Ananda is the creator and begetter of all becoming, its method is Tapas or force of the Purusha's consciousness dwelling upon its own infinite potentiality in existence and producing from it truths of conception or real Ideas, *vijñāna*, which, proceeding from an omniscient and omnipotent Self-existence, have the surety of their own fulfilment and contain in themselves the nature and law of their own becoming in the terms of mind, life and matter. The eventual omnipotence of Tapas and the infallible fulfilment of the Idea are the very foundation of all Yoga. In man we render these terms by Will and Faith,—a will that is eventually self-effective because it is of the substance of Knowledge and a faith that is the reflex in the lower consciousness of a Truth or real Idea yet unrealised in the manifestation. It is this self-certainty of the Idea which is meant by the Gita when it says, *yo yac-chraddhaḥ sa eva saḥ* , "whatever is a man's faith or the sure Idea in him, that he becomes."

We see, then, what from the psychological point of view,—and Yoga is nothing but practical psychology,—is the conception of Nature from which we have to start. It is the self-fulfilment of the Purusha through his Energy. But the movement of Nature is twofold, higher and lower, or, as we may choose to term it, divine and undivine. The distinction exists indeed for practical purposes only; for there is nothing that is not divine, and in a larger view it is as meaningless, verbally, as the distinction between natural and supernatural, for all things that are are natural. All things are in Nature and all things are in God. But, for practical purposes, there is a real distinction. The lower Nature, that which we know and are and must remain so long as the faith in us is not changed, acts through limitation and division, is of the nature of Ignorance and culminates in the life of the ego; but the higher Nature, that to which we aspire, acts by unification and transcendence of limitation, is of the nature of Knowledge and culminates in the life divine. The passage from the lower to the higher is the aim of Yoga; and this passage may effect itself by the rejection of the lower and escape into the higher,—the ordinary view-point,—or by the transformation of the lower and its elevation to the higher Nature. It is this, rather, that must be the aim of an integral Yoga.

But in either case it is always through something in the lower that we must rise into the higher existence, and the schools of Yoga each select their own point of departure or their own gate of escape. They specialise certain activities of the lower Prakriti and turn them towards the Divine. But the normal action of Nature in us is an integral movement in which the full complexity of all our elements is affected by and affects all our environments. The whole of life is the Yoga of Nature. The Yoga that we seek must also be an integral action of Nature, and the whole difference between the Yogin and the natural man will be this, that the Yogin seeks to substitute in himself for the integral action of the lower Nature working in and by ego and division the integral action of the higher Nature working in and by God and unity. If indeed our aim be only an escape from the world to God, synthesis is unnecessary and a waste of time; for then our sole practical aim must be to find out one path out of the thousand that lead to God, one shortest possible of short cuts, and not to linger exploring different paths that end in the same goal. But if our aim be a transformation of our integral being into the terms of God-existence, it is then that a synthesis becomes necessary.

The method we have to pursue, then, is to put our whole conscious being into relation and contact with the Divine and to call Him in to transform our entire being into His. Thus in a sense God Himself, the real Person in us, becomes the sadhaka of the sadhana[1] as well as the Master of the Yoga by whom the lower personality is used as the centre of a divine transfiguration and the instrument of its own perfection. In effect, the pressure of the Tapas, the force of consciousness in us dwelling in the Idea of the divine Nature upon that which we are in our entirety, produces its own realisation. The divine and all-knowing and all-effecting descends upon the limited and obscure, progressively illumines and energises the whole lower nature and substitutes its own action for all the terms of the inferior human light and mortal activity.

In psychological fact this method translates itself into the progressive surrender of the ego with its whole field and all its apparatus to the Beyond-ego with its vast and incalculable but always inevitable workings. Certainly, this is no short cut or easy sadhana. It requires a colossal faith, an absolute courage and above all an unflinching patience. For it implies three stages of which only the last can be wholly blissful or rapid,—the attempt of the ego to enter into contact with the Divine, the wide, full and therefore laborious preparation of the whole lower Nature by the divine working to receive and become the higher Nature, and the eventual transformation. In fact, however, the divine Strength, often unobserved and behind the veil, substitutes itself for our weakness and supports us through all our failings of faith, courage and patience. It "makes the blind to see and the lame to stride over the hills." The intellect becomes aware of a Law that beneficently insists and a succour that upholds; the heart speaks of a Master of all things and Friend of man or a universal Mother who upholds through all stumblings. Therefore this path is at once the most difficult imaginable and yet, in comparison with the magnitude of its effort and object, the most easy and sure of all.

There are three outstanding features of this action of the higher when it works integrally on the lower nature. In the first place it does not act according to a fixed system and succession as in the specialised methods of Yoga, but with a sort of free, scattered and yet gradually intensive and purposeful working determined by the temperament of the individual in whom it operates, the helpful materials which his nature offers and the obstacles which it presents to purification and perfection. In a sense, therefore, each man in this path has his own method of Yoga. Yet are there certain broad lines of working common to all which enable us to construct not indeed a routine system, but yet some kind of Shastra or scientific method of the synthetic Yoga.

Secondly, the process, being integral, accepts our nature such as it stands organised by our past evolution and without rejecting anything essential compels all to undergo a divine change. Everything in us is seized by the hands of a mighty Artificer and transformed into a clear image of that which it now seeks confusedly to present. In that ever-progressive experience we begin to perceive how this lower manifestation is constituted and that everything in it, however seemingly deformed or petty or vile, is the more or less distorted or imperfect figure of some element or action in the harmony of the divine Nature. We begin to understand what the Vedic Rishis meant when they spoke of the human forefathers fashioning the gods as a smith forges the crude material in his smithy.

Thirdly, the divine Power in us uses all life as the means of this integral Yoga. Every experience and outer contact with our world-environment, however trifling or however disastrous, is used for the work, and every inner experience, even to the most repellent suffering or the most humiliating fall, becomes a step on the path to perfection. And we recognise in ourselves with opened eyes the method of God in the world, His purpose of light in the obscure, of might in the weak and fallen, of delight in what is grievous and miserable. We see the divine method to be the same in the lower and in the higher working; only in the one it is pursued tardily and obscurely through the subconscious in Nature, in the other it becomes swift and self-conscious and the instrument confesses the hand of the Master. All life is a Yoga of Nature seeking to manifest God within itself. Yoga marks the stage at which this effort becomes capable of self-awareness and therefore of right completion in the individual. It is a gathering up and concentration of the movements dispersed and loosely combined in the lower evolution.

An integral method and an integral result. First, an integral realisation of Divine Being; not only a realisation of the One in its indistinguishable unity, but also in its multitude of aspects which are also necessary to the complete knowledge of it by the relative consciousness; not only realisation of unity in the Self, but of unity in the infinite diversity of activities, worlds and creatures.

Therefore, also, an integral liberation. Not only the freedom born of unbroken contact and identification of the individual being in all its parts with the Divine, *sāyujya-mukti*, by which it can become free[2] even in its separation, even in the duality; not only the *sālokya-mukti* by which the whole conscious existence dwells in the same status of being as the Divine, in the state of Sachchidananda; but also the acquisition of the divine nature by the transformation of this lower being into the human image of the Divine, *sādharmya-mukti*, and the complete and final release of all, the liberation of the consciousness from the transitory mould of the ego and its unification with the One Being, universal both in the world and the individual and transcendentally one both in the world and beyond all universe.

By this integral realisation and liberation, the perfect harmony of the results of Knowledge, Love and Works. For there is attained the complete release from ego and identification in being with the One in all and beyond all. But since the attaining consciousness is not limited by its attainment, we win also the unity in Beatitude and the harmonised diversity in Love, so that all relations of the play remain possible to us even while we retain on the heights of our being the eternal oneness with the Beloved. And by a similar wideness, being capable of a freedom in spirit that embraces life and does not depend upon withdrawal from life, we are able to become without egoism, bondage or reaction the channel in our mind and body for a divine action poured out freely upon the world.

The divine existence is of the nature not only of freedom, but of purity, beatitude and perfection. An integral purity which shall enable on the one hand the perfect reflection of the divine Being in ourselves and on the other the perfect outpouring of its Truth and Law in us in the terms of life and through the right functioning of the complex instrument we are in our outer parts, is the condition of an integral liberty. Its result is an integral beatitude, in which there becomes possible at once the Ananda of all that is in the world seen as symbols of the Divine and the Ananda of that which is not-world. And it prepares the integral perfection of our humanity as a type of the Divine in the conditions of the human manifestation, a perfection founded on a certain free universality of being, of love and joy, of play of knowledge and of play of will in power and will in unegoistic action. This integrality also can be attained by the integral Yoga.

Perfection includes perfection of mind and body, so that the highest results of Rajayoga and Hathayoga should be contained in the widest formula of the synthesis finally to be effected by mankind. At any rate a full development of the general mental and physical faculties and experiences attainable by humanity through Yoga must be included in the scope of the integral method. Nor would these have any *raison d'être* unless employed for an integral mental and physical life. Such a mental and physical life would be in its nature a translation of the spiritual existence into its right mental and physical values. Thus we would arrive at a synthesis of the three degrees of Nature and of the three modes of human existence which she has evolved or is evolving. We would include in the scope of our liberated being and perfected modes of activity the material life, our base, and the mental life, our intermediate instrument.

Nor would the integrality to which we aspire be real or even possible, if it were confined to the individual. Since our divine perfection embraces the realisation of ourselves in being, in life and in love through others as well as through ourselves, the extension of our liberty and of its results in others would be the inevitable outcome as well as the broadest utility of our liberation and perfection. And the constant and inherent attempt of such an extension would be towards its increasing and ultimately complete generalisation in mankind.

The divinising of the normal material life of man and of his great secular attempt of mental and moral self-culture in the individual and the race by this integralisation of a widely perfect spiritual existence would thus be the crown alike of our individual and of our common effort. Such a consummation being no other than the kingdom of heaven within reproduced in the kingdom of heaven without, would be also the true fulfilment of the great dream cherished in different terms by the world's religions.

The widest synthesis of perfection possible to thought is the sole effort entirely worthy of those whose dedicated vision perceives that God dwells concealed in humanity.

---

1. *Sādhana*, the practice by which perfection, *siddhi*, is attained; *sādhaka*, the Yogin who seeks by that practice the *siddhi*.
2. As the Jivanmukta, who is entirely free even without dissolution of the bodily life in a final Samadhi.

THE YOGA OF DIVINE LOVE

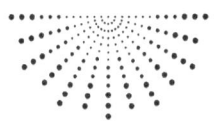

LOVE AND THE TRIPLE PATH

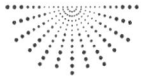

WILL, KNOWLEDGE and LOVE are the three divine powers in human nature and the life of man, and they point to the three paths by which the human soul rises to the divine. The integrality of them, the union of man with God in all the three, must therefore, as we have seen, be the foundation of an integral Yoga.

Action is the first power of life. Nature begins with force and its works which, once conscious in man, become will and its achievements; therefore it is that by turning his action Godwards the life of man best and most surely begins to become divine. It is the door of first access, the starting-point of the initiation. When the will in him is made one with the divine will and the whole action of the being proceeds from the Divine and is directed towards the Divine, the union in works is perfectly accomplished. But works fulfil themselves in knowledge; all the totality of works, says the Gita, finds its rounded culmination in knowledge, *sarvaṁ karmākhilaṁ jñāne parisamāpyate*. By union in will and works we become one in the omnipresent conscious being from whom all our will and works have their rise and draw their power and in whom they fulfil the round of their energies. And the crown of this union is love; for love is the delight of conscious union with the Being in whom we live, act and move, by whom we exist, for whom alone we learn in the end to act and to be. That is the trinity of our powers, the union of all three in God to which we arrive when we start from works as our way of access and our line of contact.

Knowledge is the foundation of a constant living in the Divine. For consciousness is the foundation of all living and being, and knowledge is the action of the consciousness, the light by which it knows itself and its realities, the power by which, starting from action, we are able to hold the inner results of thought and act in a firm growth of our conscious being until it accomplishes itself, by union, in the infinity of the divine being. The Divine meets us in many aspects and to each of them knowledge is the key, so that by knowledge we enter into and possess the infinite and divine in every way of his being, *sarvabhāvena*,[1] and receive him into us and are possessed by him in every way of ours.

Without knowledge we live blindly in him with the blindness of the power of Nature intent on its works, but forgetful of its source and possessor, undivinely therefore, deprived of the real, the full delight of our being. By knowledge arriving at conscious oneness with that which we know, — for by identity alone can complete and real knowledge exist, — the division is healed and the cause of all our limitation and discord and weakness and discontent is abolished. But knowledge is not complete without works; for the Will in being also is God and not the being or its self-aware silent existence alone, and if works find their culmination in knowledge, knowledge also finds its fulfilment in works. And, here too, love is the crown of knowledge; for love is the delight of union, and unity must be conscious of joy of union to find all the riches of its own delight. Perfect knowledge indeed leads to perfect love, integral knowledge to a rounded and multitudinous richness of love. "He who knows me" says the Gita "as the supreme Purusha," — not only as the immutable oneness, but in the many-souled movement of the divine and as that, superior to both, in which both are divinely held, — "he, because he has the integral knowledge, seeks me by love in every way of his being." This is the trinity of our powers, the union of all three in God to which we arrive when we start from knowledge.

Love is the crown of all being and its way of fulfilment, that by which it rises to all intensity and all fullness and the ecstasy of utter self-finding. For if the Being is in its very nature consciousness and by consciousness we become one with it, therefore by perfect knowledge of it fulfilled in identity, yet is delight the nature of consciousness and of the acme of delight love is the key and the secret. And if will is the power of conscious being by which it fulfils itself and by union in will we become one with the Being in its characteristic infinite power, yet all the works of that power start from delight, live in the delight, have delight for their aim and end; love of the Being in itself and in all of itself that its power of consciousness manifests, is the way to the perfect wideness of the Ananda. Love is the power and passion of the divine self-delight and without love we may get the rapt peace of its infinity, the absorbed silence of the Ananda, but not its absolute depth of richness and fullness. Love leads us from the suffering of division into the bliss of perfect union, but without losing that joy of the act of union which is the soul's greatest discovery and for which the life of the cosmos is a long preparation. Therefore to approach God by love is to prepare oneself for the greatest possible spiritual fulfilment.

Love fulfilled does not exclude knowledge, but itself brings knowledge; and the completer the knowledge, the richer the possibility of love. "By Bhakti" says the Lord in the Gita "shall a man know Me in all my extent and greatness and as I am in the principles of my being, and when he has known Me in the principles of my being, then he enters into Me." Love without knowledge is a passionate and intense, but blind, crude, often dangerous thing, a great power, but also a stumbling-block; love, limited in knowledge, condemns itself in its fervour and often by its very fervour to narrowness; but love leading to perfect knowledge brings the infinite and absolute union. Such love is not inconsistent with, but rather throws itself with joy into divine works; for it loves God and is one with him in all his being, and therefore in all beings, and to work for the world is then to feel and fulfil multitudinously one's love for God. This is the trinity of our powers, the union of all three in God to which we arrive when we start on our journey by the path of devotion with Love for the Angel of the Way to find in the ecstasy of the divine delight of the All-Lover's being the fulfilment of ours, its secure home and blissful abiding-place and the centre of its universal radiation.

Since then in the union of these three powers lies our base of perfection, the seeker of an integral self-fulfilment in the Divine must avoid or throw away, if he has them at all, the misunderstanding and mutual depreciation which we often find existent between the followers of the three paths. Those who have the cult of knowledge seem often, if not to despise, yet to look downward from their dizzy eminence on the path of the devotee as if it were a thing inferior, ignorant, good only for souls that are not yet ready for the heights of the Truth. It is true that devotion without knowledge is often a thing raw, crude, blind and dangerous, as the errors, crimes, follies of the religious have too often shown. But this is because devotion in them has not found its own path, its own real principle, has not therefore really entered on the path, but is fumbling and feeling after it, is on one of the bypaths that lead to it; and knowledge too at this stage is as imperfect as devotion, dogmatic, schismatic, intolerant, bound up in the narrowness of some single and exclusive principle, even that being usually very imperfectly seized. When the devotee has grasped the power that shall raise him, has really laid hold on love, that in the end purifies and enlarges him as effectively as knowledge can; they are equal powers, though their methods of arriving at the same goal are different. The pride of the philosopher looking down on the passion of the devotee arises, as does all pride, from a certain deficiency of his nature; for the intellect too exclusively developed misses what the heart has to offer. The intellect is not in every way superior to the heart; if it opens more readily doors at which the heart is apt to fumble in vain, it is, itself, apt to miss truths which to the heart are very near and easy to hold. And if when the way of thought deepens into spiritual experience, it arrives readily at the etherial heights, pinnacles, skiey widenesses, it cannot without the aid of the heart fathom the intense and rich abysses and oceanic depths of the divine being and the divine Ananda.

The way of Bhakti is supposed often to be necessarily inferior because it proceeds by worship which belongs to that stage of spiritual experience where there is a difference, an insufficient unity between the human soul and the Divine, because its very principle is love and love means always two, the lover and the beloved, a dualism therefore, while oneness is the highest spiritual experience, and because it seeks after the personal God while the Impersonal is the highest and the eternal truth, if not even the sole Reality. But worship is only the first step on the path of devotion. Where external worship changes into the inner adoration, real

Bhakti begins; that deepens into the intensity of divine love; that love leads to the joy of closeness in our relations with the Divine; the joy of closeness passes into the bliss of union. Love too as well as knowledge brings us to a highest oneness and it gives to that oneness its greatest possible depth and intensity. It is true that love returns gladly upon a difference in oneness, by which the oneness itself becomes richer and sweeter. But here we may say that the heart is wiser than the thought, at least than that thought which fixes upon opposite ideas of the Divine and concentrates on one to the exclusion of the other which seems its contrary, but is really its complement and a means of its greatest fulfilment. This is the weakness of the mind that it limits itself by its thoughts, its positive and negative ideas, the aspects of the Divine Reality that it sees, and tends too much to pit one against the other.

Thought in the mind, *vicāra*, the philosophic trend by which mental knowledge approaches the Divine, is apt to lend a greater importance to the abstract over the concrete, to that which is high and remote over that which is intimate and near. It finds a greater truth in the delight of the One in itself, a lesser truth or even a falsehood in the delight of the One in the Many and of the Many in the One, a greater truth in the impersonal and the Nirguna, a lesser truth or a falsehood in the personal and the Saguna. But the Divine is beyond our oppositions of ideas, beyond the logical contradictions we make between his aspects. He is not, we have seen, bound and restricted by exclusive unity; his oneness realises itself in infinite variation and to the joy of that love has the completest key, without therefore missing the joy of the unity. The highest knowledge and highest spiritual experience by knowledge find his oneness as perfect in his various relations with the Many as in his self-absorbed delight. If to thought the Impersonal seems the wider and higher truth, the Personal a narrower experience, the spirit finds both of them to be aspects of a Reality which figures itself in both, and if there is a knowledge of that Reality to which thought arrives by insistence on the infinite Impersonality, there is also a knowledge of it to which love arrives by insistence on the infinite Personality. The spiritual experience of each leads, if followed to the end, to the same ultimate Truth. By Bhakti as by knowledge, as the Gita tells us, we arrive at unity with the Purushottama, the Supreme who contains in himself the impersonal and numberless personalities, the qualitiless and infinite qualities, pure being, consciousness and delight and the endless play of their relations.

The devotee on the other hand tends to look down on the sawdust dryness of mere knowledge. And it is true that philosophy by itself without the rapture of spiritual experience is something as dry as it is clear and cannot give all the satisfaction we seek, that its spiritual experience even, when it has not left its supports of thought and shot up beyond the mind, lives too much in an abstract delight and that what it reaches, is not indeed the void it seems to the passion of the heart, but still has the limitations of the peaks. On the other hand, love itself is no complete without knowledge. The Gita distinguishes between three initial kinds of Bhakti, that which seeks refuge in the Divine from the sorrows of the world, *ārta*, that which, desiring, approaches the Divine as the giver of its good, *arthārthī*, and that which attracted by what it already loves, but does not yet know, yearns to know this divine Unknown, *jijñāsu*; but it gives the palm to the Bhakti that knows. Evidently the intensity of passion which says, "I do not understand, I love," and, loving, cares not to understand, is not love's last self-expression, but its first, nor is it its highest intensity. Rather as knowledge of the Divine grows, delight in the Divine and love of it must increase. Nor can mere rapture be secure without the foundation of knowledge; to live in what we love, gives that security, and to live in it means to be one with it in consciousness, and oneness of consciousness is the perfect condition of knowledge. Knowledge of the Divine gives to love of the Divine its firmest security, opens to it its own widest joy of experience, raises it to its highest pinnacles of outlook.

If the mutual misunderstandings of these two powers are an ignorance, no less so is the tendency of both to look down on the way of works as inferior to their own loftier pitch of spiritual achievement. There is an intensity of love, as there is an intensity of knowledge, to which works seem something outward and distracting. But works are only thus outward and distracting when we have not found oneness of will and consciousness with the Supreme. When once that is found, works become the very power of knowledge and the very outpouring of love. If knowledge is the very state of oneness and love its bliss, divine works are the living power of its light and sweetness. There is a movement of love, as in the aspiration of human love, to separate the lover and the loved in the enjoyment of their exclusive oneness away from the world and from all others, shut up in the nuptial chambers of the heart. That is perhaps an inevitable movement of this path. But still the widest love fulfilled in knowledge sees the world not as something other and hostile to this joy, but as the being of the Beloved and all creatures as his being, and in that vision divine works find their joy and their justification.

This is the knowledge in which an integral Yoga must live. We have to start Godward from the powers of the mind, the intellect, the will, the heart, and in the mind all is limited. Limitations, exclusiveness there can hardly fail to be at the beginning and for a long time on the way. But an integral Yoga will wear these more loosely than more exclusive ways of seeking, and it will sooner emerge from the mental necessity. It may commence with the way of love, as with the way of knowledge or of works; but where they meet, is the beginning of its joy of fulfilment. Love it cannot miss, even if it does not start from it; for love is the crown of works and the flowering of knowledge.

---

1. Gita.

THE MOTIVES OF DEVOTION

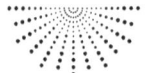

ALL RELIGION begins with the conception of some Power or existence greater and higher than our limited and mortal selves, a thought and act of worship done to that Power, and an obedience offered to its will, its laws or its demands. But Religion, in its beginnings, sets an immeasurable gulf between the Power thus conceived, worshipped and obeyed and the worshipper. Yoga in its culmination abolishes the gulf; for Yoga is union. We arrive at union with it through knowledge; for as our first obscure conceptions of it clarify, enlarge, deepen, we come to recognise it as our own highest self, the origin and sustainer of our being and that towards which it tends. We arrive at union with it through works; for from simply obeying we come to identify our will with its Will, since only in proportion as it is identified with this Power that is its source and ideal, can our will become perfect and divine. We arrive at union with it also by worship; for the thought and act of a distant worship develops into the necessity of close adoration and this into the intimacy of love, and the consummation of love is union with the Beloved. It is from this development of worship that the Yoga of devotion starts and it is by this union with the Beloved that it finds its highest point and consummation.

All our instincts and the movements of our being begin by supporting themselves on the ordinary motives of our lower human nature, — mixed and egoistic motives at first, but afterwards they purify and elevate themselves, they become an intense and special need of our higher nature quite apart from the results our actions bring with them; finally they exalt themselves into a sort of categorical imperative of our being, and it is through our obedience to this that we arrive at that supreme something self-existent in us which was all the time drawing us towards it, first by the lures of our egoistic nature, then by something much higher, larger, more universal, until we are able to feel its own direct attraction which is the strongest and most imperative of all. In the transformation of ordinary religious worship into the Yoga of pure Bhakti we see this development from the motived and interested worship of popular religion into a principle of motiveless and self-existent love. This last is in fact the touchstone of the real Bhakti and shows whether we are really in the central way or are only upon one of the bypaths leading to it. We have to throw away the props of our weakness, the motives of the ego, the lures of our lower nature before we can deserve the divine union.

Faced with the sense of a Power or perhaps a number of Powers greater and higher than himself by whom his life in Nature is overshadowed, influenced, governed, man naturally applies to it or to them the first primitive feelings of the natural being among the difficulties, desires and dangers of that life, — fear and interest. The enormous part played by these motives in the evolution of the religious instinct, is undeniable, and in fact, man being what he is, it could hardly have been less; and even when religion has advanced fairly far on its road, we see these motives still surviving, active, playing a sufficiently large part, justified and appealed to by Religion herself in support of her claims on man. The fear of God, it is said, — or, it may be added for the sake of historical truth, the fear of the Gods, — is the beginning of religion, a half-truth upon which scientific research, trying to trace the evolution of religion, ordinarily in a critical and often a hostile rather than in a sympathetic spirit, has laid undue emphasis. But not the fear of God only, for man does not act, even most primitively, from fear alone, but from twin motives, fear and desire, fear of things unpleasant and maleficent and desire of things pleasant and beneficent, — therefore from fear and interest. Life to him is primarily and engrossingly, — until he learns to live more in his soul and only secondarily in the action and reaction of outward things, — a series of actions and results, things to be desired, pursued and gained by action and things to be dreaded and shunned, yet which may come upon him as a result of action. And it is not only by his own action but by that also of others and of Nature around him that these things come to him. As soon, then, as he comes to sense a Power behind all this which can influence or determine action and result, he conceives of it as a dispenser of boons and sufferings, able and under certain conditions willing to help him or hurt, save and destroy.

In the most primitive parts of his being he conceives of it as a thing of natural egoistic impulses like himself, beneficent when pleased, maleficent when offended; worship is then a means of propitiation by gifts and a supplication by prayer. He gets God on his side by praying to him and flattering him. With a more advanced mentality, he conceives of the action of life as reposing on a certain principle of divine justice, which he reads always according to his own ideas and character, as a sort of enlarged copy of his human justice; he conceives the idea of moral good and evil and looks upon suffering and calamity and all things unpleasant as a punishment for his sins and upon happiness and good fortune and all things pleasant as a reward of his virtue. God appears to him as a king, judge, legislator, executor of justice. But still regarding him as a sort of magnified Man, he imagines that as his own justice can be deflected by prayers and propitiation, so the divine justice can also be deflected by the same means. Justice is to him reward and punishment, and the justice of punishment can be modified by mercy to the suppliant, while rewards can be supplemented by special favours and kindness such as Power when pleased can always bestow on its adherents and worshippers. Moreover God like ourselves is capable of wrath and revenge, and wrath and revenge can be turned by gifts and supplication and atonement; he is capable too of partiality, and his partiality can be attracted by gifts, by prayer and by praise. Therefore instead of relying solely on the observation of the moral law, worship as prayer and propitiation is still continued.

Along with these motives there arises another development of personal feeling, first of the awe which one naturally feels for something vast, powerful and incalculable beyond our nature by a certain inscrutability in the springs and extent of its action, and of the veneration and adoration which one feels for that which is higher in its nature or its perfection than ourselves. For, even while preserving largely the idea of a God endowed with the qualities of human nature, there still grows up along with it, mixed up with it or superadded, the conception of an omniscience, an omnipotence and a mysterious perfection quite other than our nature. A confused mixture of all these motives, variously developed, often modified, subtilised or glossed over, is what constitutes nine tenths of popular religion; the other tenth is a suffusion of the rest by the percolation into it of nobler, more beautiful and profounder ideas of the Divine which minds of a greater spirituality have been able to bring into the more primitive religious concepts of mankind. The result is usually crude enough and a ready target for the shafts of scepticism and unbelief, — powers of the human mind which have their utility even for faith and religion, since they compel a religion to purify gradually what is crude or false in its conceptions. But what we have to see is how far in purifying and elevating the religious instinct of worship any of these earlier motives need to survive and enter into the Yoga of devotion which itself starts from worship. That depends on how far they correspond to any truth of the divine Being and its relations with the human soul; for we seek by Bhakti union with the Divine and true relation with it, with its truth and not with any mirage of our lower nature and of its egoistic impulses and ignorant conceptions.

The ground on which sceptical unbelief assails Religion, namely, that there is in fact no conscient Power or Being in the universe greater and higher than ourselves or in any way influencing or controlling our existence, is one which Yoga cannot accept, as that would contradict all spiritual experience and make Yoga itself impossible. Yoga is not a matter of theory or dogma, like philosophy or popular religion, but a matter of experience. Its experience is that of a conscient universal and supracosmic Being with whom it brings us into union, and this conscious experience of union with the Invisible, always renewable and verifiable, is as valid as our conscious experience of a physical world and of visible bodies with whose invisible minds we daily communicate. Yoga proceeds by conscious union, the conscious being is its instrument, and a conscious union with the Inconscient cannot be. It is true that it goes beyond the human consciousness and in Samadhi becomes superconscient, but this is not an annullation of our conscious being, it is only its self-exceeding, the going beyond its present level and normal limits.

So far, then, all Yogic experience is agreed. But Religion and the Yoga of Bhakti go farther; they attribute to this Being a Personality and human relations with the human being. In both the human being approaches the Divine by means of his humanity, with human emotions, as he would approach a fellowbeing, but with more intense and exalted feelings; and not only so, but the Divine also responds in a manner answering to these emotions. In that possibility of response lies the whole question; for if the Divine is impersonal, featureless and relationless, no such response is possible and all human approach to it becomes an absurdity; we must rather dehumanise, depersonalise, annul ourselves in so far as we are human beings or any kind of beings; on no other conditions and by no other means can we approach it. Love, fear, prayer, praise, worship of an Impersonality which has no relation with us or with anything in the universe and no feature that our minds can lay hold of, are obviously an irrational foolishness. On such terms religion and devotion become out of the question. The Adwaitin in order to find a religious basis for his bare and sterile philosophy, has to admit the practical existence of God and the gods and to delude his mind with the language of Maya. Buddhism only became a popular religion when Buddha had taken the place of the supreme Deity as an object of worship.

Even if the Supreme be capable of relations with us but only of impersonal relations, religion is robbed of its human vitality and the Path of Devotion ceases to be effective or even possible. We may indeed apply our human emotions to it, but in a vague and imprecise fashion, with no hope of a human response: the only way in which it can respond to us, is by stilling our emotions and throwing upon us its own impersonal calm and immutable equality; and this is what in fact happens when we approach the pure impersonality of the Godhead. We can obey it as a Law, lift our souls to it in aspiration towards its tranquil being, grow into it by shedding from us our emotional nature; the human being in us is not satisfied, but it is quieted, balanced, stilled. But the Yoga of devotion, agreeing in this with Religion, insists on a closer and warmer worship than this impersonal aspiration. It aims at a divine fulfilment of the humanity in us as well as of the impersonal part of our being; it aims at a divine satisfaction of the emotional being of man. It demands of the Supreme acceptance of our love and a response in kind; as we delight in Him and seek Him, so it believes that He too delights in us and seeks us. Nor can this demand be condemned as irrational, for if the supreme and universal Being did not take any delight in us, it is not easy to see how we could have come into being or could remain in being, and if He does not at all draw us towards him, — a divine seeking of us, — there would seem to be no reason in Nature why we should turn from the round of our normal existence to seek Him.

Therefore that there may be at all any possibility of a Yoga of devotion, we must assume first that the supreme Existence is not an abstraction or a state of existence, but a conscious Being; secondly, that he meets us in the universe and is in some way immanent in it as well as its source,—otherwise, we should have to go out of cosmic life to meet him; thirdly, that he is capable of personal relations with us and must therefore be not incapable of personality; finally, that when we approach him by our human emotions, we receive a response in kind. This does not mean that the nature of the Divine is precisely the same as our human nature though upon a larger scale, or that it is that nature pure of certain perversions and God a magnified or else an ideal Man. God is not and cannot be an ego limited by his qualities as we are in our normal consciousness. But on the other hand our human consciousness must certainly originate and have been derived from the Divine; though the forms which it takes in us may and must be other than the divine because we are limited by ego, not universal, not superior to our nature, not greater than our qualities and their workings, as he is, still our human emotions and impulses must have behind them a Truth in him of which they are the limited and very often, therefore, the perverse or even the degraded forms. By approaching him through our emotional being we approach that Truth, it comes down to us to meet our emotions and lift them towards it; through it our emotional being is united with him.

Secondly, this supreme Being is also the universal Being and our relations with the universe are all means by which we are prepared for entering into relation with him. All the emotions with which we confront the action of the universal existence upon us, are really directed towards him, in ignorance at first, but it is by directing them in growing knowledge towards him that we enter into more intimate relations with him, and all that is false and ignorant in them will fall away as we draw nearer towards unity. To all of them he answers, taking us in the stage of progress in which we are; for if we met no kind of response or help to our imperfect approach, the more perfect relations could never be established. Even as men approach him, so he accepts them and responds too by the divine Love to their bhakti, *tathaiva bhajate*. Whatever form of being, whatever qualities they lend to him, through that form and those qualities he helps them to develop, encourages or governs their advance and in their straight way or their crooked draws them towards him. What they see of him is a truth, but a truth represented to them in the terms of their own being and consciousness, partially, distortedly, not in the terms of its own higher reality, not in the aspect which it assumes when we become aware of the complete Divinity. This is the justification of the cruder and more primitive elements of religion and also their sentence of transience and passing. They are justified because there is a truth of the Divine behind them and only so could that truth of the Divine be approached in that stage of the developing human consciousness and be helped forward; they are condemned, because to persist always in these crude conceptions and relations with the Divine is to miss that closer union towards which these crude beginnings are the first steps, however faltering.

All life, we have said, is a Yoga of Nature; here in this material world life is her reaching out from her first inconscience towards a return to union with the conscient Divine from whom she proceeded. In religion the mind of man, her accomplished instrument, becomes aware of her goal in him, responds to her aspiration. Even popular religion is a sort of ignorant Yoga of devotion. But it does not become what we specifically call Yoga until the motive becomes in a certain degree clairvoyant, until it sees that union is its object and that love is the principle of union, and until therefore it tries to realise love and lose its separative character in love. When that has been accomplished, then the Yoga has taken its decisive step and is sure of its fruition. Thus the motives of devotion have first to direct themselves engrossingly and predominantly towards the Divine, then to transform themselves so that they are rid of their more earthy elements and finally to take their stand in pure and perfect love. All those that cannot coexist with the perfect union of love, must eventually fall away, while only those that can form themselves into expressions of divine love and into means of enjoying divine love, can remain. For love is the one emotion in us which can be entirely motiveless and self-existent; love need have no other motive than love. For all our emotions arise either from the seeking after delight and the possession of it, or from the baffling of the search, or from the failure of the delight we have possessed or had thought to grasp; but love is that by which we can enter directly into possession of the self-existent delight of the divine Being. Divine love is indeed itself that possession and, as it were, the body of the Ananda.

These are the truths which condition our approach to this Yoga and our journey on this path. There are subsidiary questions which arise and trouble the intellect of man, but, though we may have yet to deal with them they are not essential. Yoga of Bhakti is a matter of the heart and not of the intellect. For even for the knowledge which comes on this way, we set out from the heart and not from the intelligence. The truth of the motives of the heart's devotion and their final arrival and in some sort their disappearance into the supreme and unique self-existent motive of love, is therefore all that initially and essentially concerns us. Such difficult questions there are as whether the Divine has an original supraphysical form or power of form from which all forms proceed or is eternally formless; all we need at present say is that the Divine does at least accept the various forms which the devotee gives to him and through them meets him in love, while the mixing of our spirits with his spirit is essential to the fruition of Bhakti. So too, certain religions and religious philosophies seek to bind down devotion by a conception of an eternal difference between the human soul and the Divine, without which they say love and devotion cannot exist, while that philosophy which considers that One alone exists, consigns love and devotion to a movement in the ignorance, necessary perhaps or at the least useful as a preparatory movement while yet the ignorance lasts, but impossible when all difference is abolished and therefore to be transcended and discarded. We may hold, however, the truth of the one existence in this sense that all in Nature is the Divine even though God be more than all in Nature, and love becomes then a movement by which the Divine in Nature and man takes possession of and enjoys the delight of the universal and the supreme Divine. In any case, love has necessarily a twofold fulfilment by its very nature, that by which the lover and the beloved enjoy their union in difference and all too that enhances the joy of various union, and that by which they throw themselves into each other and become one Self. That truth is quite sufficient to start with, for it is the very nature of love, and since love is the essential motive of this Yoga, as is the whole nature of love, so will be too the crown and fulfilment of the movement of the Yoga.

THE GODWARD EMOTIONS

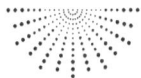

THE PRINCIPLE OF YOGA is to turn Godward all or any of the powers of the human consciousness so that through that activity of the being there may be contact, relation, union. In the Yoga of Bhakti it is the emotional nature that is made the instrument. Its main principle is to adopt some human relation between man and the Divine Being by which through the ever intenser flowing of the heart's emotions towards him the human soul may at last be wedded to and grow one with him in a passion of divine Love. It is not ultimately the pure peace of oneness or the power and desireless will of oneness, but the ecstatic joy of union which the devotee seeks by his Yoga. Every feeling that can make the heart ready for this ecstasy the Yoga admits; everything that detracts from it must increasingly drop away as the strong union of love becomes closer and more perfect.

All the feelings with which religion approaches the worship, service and love of God, the Yoga admits, if not as its final accompaniments, yet as preparatory movements of the emotional nature. But there is one feeling with which the Yoga, at least as practised in India, has very little dealing. In certain religions, in most perhaps, the idea of the fear of God plays a very large part, sometimes the largest, and the Godfearing man is the typical worshipper of these religions. The sentiment of fear is indeed perfectly consistent with devotion of a certain kind and up to a certain point; at its highest it rises into a worship of the divine Power, the divine Justice, divine Law, divine Righteousness, and ethical obedience, an awed reverence for the almighty Creator and Judge. Its motive is therefore ethico-religious and it belongs not so strictly to the devotee, but to the man of works moved by a devotion to the divine ordainer and judge of his works. It regards God as the King and does not approach too near the glory of his throne unless justified by righteousness or led there by a mediator who will turn away the divine wrath for sin. Even when it draws nearest, it keeps an awed distance between itself and the high object of its worship. It cannot embrace the Divine with all the fearless confidence of the child in his mother or of the lover in his beloved or with that intimate sense of oneness which perfect love brings with it.

The origin of this divine fear was crude enough in some of the primitive popular religions. It was the perception of powers in the world greater than man, obscure in their nature and workings, which seemed always ready to strike him down in his prosperity and to smite him for any actions which displeased them. Fear of the gods arose from man's ignorance of God and his ignorance of the laws that govern the world. It attributed to the higher powers caprice and human passion; it made them in the image of the great ones of the earth, capable of whim, tyranny, personal enmity, jealous of any greatness in man which might raise him above the littleness of terrestrial nature and bring him too near to the divine nature. With such notions no real devotion could arise, except that doubtful kind which the weaker may feel for the stronger whose protection he can buy by worship and gifts and propitiation and obedience to such laws as he may have laid upon those beneath him and may enforce by rewards and punishments, or else the submissive and prostrate reverence and adoration which one may feel for a greatness, glory, wisdom, sovereign power which is above the world and is the source or at any rate the regulator of all its laws and happenings.

A nearer approach to the beginnings of the way of devotion becomes possible when this element of divine Power disengages itself from these crudities and fixes on the idea of a divine ruler, creator of the world and master of the Law who governs the earth and heavens and is the guide and helper and saviour of his creatures. This larger and higher idea of the divine Being long kept many elements and still keeps some elements of the old crudity. The Jews who brought it forward most prominently and from whom it overspread a great part of the world, could believe in a God of righteousness who was exclusive, arbitrary, wrathful, jealous, often cruel and even wantonly sanguinary. Even now it is possible for some to believe in a Creator who has made heaven and hell, an eternal hell, the two poles of his creation, and has even according to some religions predestined the souls he has created not only to sin and punishment, but to an eternal damnation. But even apart from these extravagances of a childish religious belief, the idea of the almighty Judge, Legislator, King, is a crude and imperfect idea of the Divine, when taken by itself, because it takes an inferior and an external truth for the main truth and it tends to prevent a higher approach to a more intimate reality. It exaggerates the importance of the sense of sin and thereby prolongs and increases the soul's fear and self-distrust and weakness. It attaches the pursuit of virtue and the shunning of sin to the idea of rewards and punishment, though given in an after life, and makes them dependent on the lower motives of fear and interest instead of the higher spirit which should govern the ethical being. It makes hell and heaven and not the Divine himself the object of the human soul in its religious living. These crudities have served their turn in the slow education of the human mind, but they are of no utility to the Yogin who knows that whatever truth they may represent belongs rather to the external relations of the developing human soul with the external law of the universe than any intimate truth of the inner relations of the human soul with the Divine; but it is these which are the proper field of Yoga.

Still out of this conception there arise certain developments which bring us nearer to the threshold of the Yoga of devotion. First, there can emerge the idea of the Divine as the source and law and aim of our ethical being and from this there can come the knowledge of him as the highest Self to which our active nature aspires, the Will to which we have to assimilate our will, the eternal Right and Purity and Truth and Wisdom into harmony with which our nature has to grow and towards whose being our being is attracted. By this way we arrive at the Yoga of works, and this Yoga has a place for personal devotion to the Divine, for the divine Will appears as the Master of our works to whose voice we must listen, whose divine impulsion we must obey and whose work it is the sole business of our active life and will to do. Secondly, there emerges the idea of the divine Spirit, the father of all who extends his wings of benignant protection and love over all his creatures, and from that grows between the soul and the Divine the relation of father and child, a relation of love, and as a result the relation of brotherhood with our fellow-beings. These relations of the Divine into the calm pure light of whose nature we have to grow and the Master whom we approach through works and service, the Father who responds to the love of the soul that approaches him as the child, are admitted elements of the Yoga of devotion.

The moment we come well into these developments and their deeper spiritual meaning, the motive of the fear of God becomes otiose, superfluous and even impossible. It is of importance chiefly in the ethical field when the soul has not yet grown sufficiently to follow good for its own sake and needs an authority above it whose wrath or whose stern passionless judgment it can fear and found upon that fear its fidelity to virtue. When we grow into spirituality, this motive can no longer remain except by the lingering on of some confusion in the mind, some persistence of the old mentality. Moreover, the ethical aim in Yoga is different from that of the external idea of virtue. Ordinarily, ethics is regarded as a sort of machinery of right action, the act is everything and how to do the right act is the whole question and the whole trouble. But to the Yogin action is chiefly important not for its own sake, but rather as a means for the growth of the soul Godward. Therefore what Indian spiritual writings lay stress upon is not so much the quality of the action to be done as the quality of the soul from which the action flows, upon its truth, fearlessness, purity, love, compassion, benevolence, absence of the will to hurt, and upon the actions as their outflowings. The old western idea that human nature is intrinsically bad and virtue is a thing to be followed out in despite of our fallen nature to which it is contrary, is foreign to the Indian mentality trained from ancient times in the ideas of the Yogins. Our nature contains, as well as its passionate rajasic and its downward-tending tamasic quality, a purer sattwic element and it is the encouragement of this, its highest part, which is the business of ethics. By it we increase the divine nature, *daivī prakṛti*, which is present in us and get rid of the Titanic and demoniac elements. Not therefore the Hebraic righteousness of the Godfearing man, but the purity, love, beneficence, truth, fearlessness, harmlessness of the saint and the God-lover are the goal of the ethical growth according to this notion. And, speaking more largely, to grow into the divine nature is the consummation of the ethical being. This can be done best by realising God as the higher Self, the guiding and uplifting Will or the Master whom we love and serve. Not fear of him, but love of him and aspiration to the freedom and eternal purity of his being must be the motive.

Certainly, fear enters into the relations of the master and the servant and even of the father and the child, but only when they are on the human level, when control and subjection and punishment figure predominantly in them and love is obliged to efface itself more or less behind the mask of authority. The Divine even as the Master does not punish anybody, does not threaten, does not force obedience. It is the human soul that has freely to come to the Divine and offer itself to his overpowering force that he may seize and uplift it towards his own divine levels, and give it that joy of mastery of the finite nature by the Infinite and of service to the Highest by which there comes freedom from the ego and the lower nature. Love is the key of this relation, and this service, *dāsyam*, is in Indian Yoga the happy service of the divine Friend or the passionate service to the divine Beloved. The Master of the worlds who in the Gita demands of his servant, the bhakta, to be nothing more in life than his instrument, makes this claim as the friend, the guide, the higher Self, and describes himself as the Lord of all the worlds who is the friend of all creatures, *sarvalokamaheśvaraṁ suhṛdaṁ sarvabhūtānām*; the two relations in fact must go together and neither can be perfect without the other. So too it is not the fatherhood of God as the Creator who demands obedience because he is the maker of our being, but the fatherhood of love which leads us towards the closer soul-union of Yoga. Love is the real key in both, and perfect love is inconsistent with the admission of the motive of fear. Closeness of the human soul to the Divine is the object, and fear sets always a barrier and a distance; even awe and reverence for the divine Power are a sign of distance and division and they disappear in the intimacy of the union of love. Moreover, fear belongs to the lower nature, to the lower self, and in approaching the higher Self must be put aside before we can enter into its presence.

This relation of the divine fatherhood and the closer relation with the Divine as the Mother-Soul of the universe have their springs in another early religious motive. One type of the Bhakta, says the Gita, is the devotee who comes to the Divine as the giver of his wants, the giver of his good, the satisfier of the needs of his inner and his outer being. "I bring to my bhakta" says the Lord "his getting and his having of good, *yogakṣemaṁ vahāmyaham.*" The life of man is a life of wants and needs and therefore of desires, not only in his physical and vital, but in his mental and spiritual being. When he becomes conscious of a greater Power governing the world, he approaches it through prayer for the fulfilment of his needs, for help in his rough journey, for protection and aid in his struggle. Whatever crudities there may be in the ordinary religious approach to God by prayer, and there are many, especially that attitude which imagines the Divine as if capable of being propitiated, bribed, flattered into acquiescence or indulgence by praise, entreaty and gifts and has often little regard to the spirit in which he is approached, still this way of turning to the Divine is an essential movement of our religious being and reposes on a universal truth.

The efficacy of prayer is often doubted and prayer itself supposed to be a thing irrational and necessarily superfluous and ineffective. It is true that the universal will executes always its aim and cannot be deflected by egoistic propitiation and entreaty, it is true of the Transcendent who expresses himself in the universal order that being omniscient his larger knowledge must foresee the thing to be done and it does not need direction or stimulation by human thought and that the individual's desires are not and cannot be in any world-order the true determining factor. But neither is that order or the execution of the universal will altogether effected by mechanical Law, but by powers and forces of which for human life at least human will, aspiration and faith are not among the least important. Prayer is only a particular form given to that will, aspiration and faith. Its forms are very often crude and not only childlike, which is in itself no defect, but childish; but still it has a real power and significance. Its power and sense is to put the will, aspiration and faith of man into touch with the divine Will as that of a conscious Being with whom we can enter into conscious and living relations. For our will and aspiration can act either by our own strength and endeavour, which can no doubt be made a thing great and effective whether for lower or higher purposes, — and there are plenty of disciplines which put it forward as the one force to be used, — or it can act in dependence upon and with subordination to the divine or the universal Will. And this latter way again may either look upon that Will as responsive indeed to our aspiration, but almost mechanically, by a sort of law of energy, or at any rate quite impersonaly, or else it may look upon it as responding consciously to the divine aspiration and faith of the human soul and consciously bringing to it the help, the guidance, the protection and fruition demanded, *yogakṣemaṁ vahāmyaham*.

Prayer helps to prepare this relation for us at first on the lower plane even while it is there consistent with much that is mere egoism and self-delusion; but afterwards we can draw towards the spiritual truth which is behind it. It is not then the giving of the thing asked for that matters, but the relation itself, the contact of man's life with God, the conscious interchange. In spiritual matters and in the seeking of spiritual gains, this conscious relation is a great power; it is a much greater power than our own entirely self-reliant struggle and effort and it brings a fuller spiritual growth and experience. Necessarily in the end prayer either ceases in the greater thing for which it prepared us, — in fact the form we call prayer is not itself essential so long as the faith, the will, the aspiration are there, — or remains only for the joy of the relation. Also its objects, the *artha* or interest it seeks to realise, become higher and higher until we reach the highest motiveless devotion, which is that of divine love pure and simple without any other demand or longing.

The relations which arise out of this attitude towards the Divine, are that of the divine Father and the Mother with the child and that of the divine Friend. To the Divine as these things the human soul comes for help, for protection, for guidance, for fruition, — or if knowledge be the aim, to the Guide, Teacher, Giver of light, for the Divine is the Sun of knowledge, — or it comes in pain and suffering for relief and solace and deliverance, it may be deliverance either from the suffering itself or from the world-existence which is the habitat of the suffering or from all its inner and real causes.[1] In these things we find there is a certain gradation. For the relation of fatherhood is always less close, intense, passionate, intimate, and therefore it is less resorted to in the Yoga which seeks for the closest union. That of the divine Friend is a thing sweeter and more intimate, admits of an equality and intimacy even in inequality and the beginning of mutual self-giving; at its closest when all idea of other giving and taking disappears, when this relation becomes motiveless except for the one sole all-sufficing motive of love, it turns into the free and happy relation of the playmate in the Lila of existence. But closer and more intimate still is the relation of the Mother and the child, and that therefore plays a very large part wherever the religious impulse is most richly fervent and springs most warmly from the heart of man. The soul goes to the Mother-Soul in all its desires and troubles and the divine Mother wishes that it should be so, so that she may pour out her heart of love. It turns to her too because of the self-existent nature of this love and because that points us to the home towards which we turn from our wanderings in the world and to the bosom in which we find our rest.

But the highest and the greatest relation is that which starts from none of the ordinary religious motives, but is rather of the very essence of Yoga, springs from the very nature of love itself; it is the passion of the Lover and the Beloved. Wherever there is the desire of the soul for its utter union with God, this form of the divine yearning makes its way even into religions which seem to do without it and give it no place in their ordinary system. Here the one thing asked for is love, the one thing feared is the loss of love, the one sorrow is the sorrow of separation of love; for all other things either do not exist for the lover or come in only as incidents or as results and not as objects or conditions of love. All love is indeed in its nature self-existent because it springs from a secret oneness in being and a sense of that oneness or desire of oneness in the heart between souls that are yet able to conceive of themselves as different from each other and divided. Therefore all these other relations too can arrive at their self-existent motiveless joy of being for the sake of love alone. But still they start from and to the end they to some extent find a satisfaction of their play in other motives. But here the beginning is love and the end is love and the whole aim is love. There is indeed the desire of possession, but even this is overcome in the fullness of the self-existent love and the final demand of the Bhakta is simply that his bhakti may never cease nor diminish. He does not ask for heaven or for liberation from birth or for any other object, but only that his love may be eternal and absolute.

Love is a passion and it seeks for two things, eternity and intensity, and in the relation of the Lover and Beloved the seeking for eternity and for intensity is instinctive and self-born. Love is a seeking for mutual possession, and it is here that the demand for mutual possession becomes absolute. Passing beyond desire of possession which means a difference, it is a seeking for oneness, and it is here that the idea of oneness, of two souls merging into each other and becoming one finds the acme of its longing and the utterness of its satisfaction. Love, too, is a yearning for beauty, and it is here that the yearning is eternally satisfied in the vision and the touch and the joy of the All-beautiful. Love is a child and a seeker of Delight, and it is here that it finds the highest possible ecstasy both of the heart-consciousness and of every fibre of the being. Moreover, this relation is that which as between human being and human being demands the most and, even while reaching the greatest intensities, is still the least satisfied, because only in the Divine can it find its real and its utter satisfaction. Therefore it is here most that the turning of human emotion Godwards finds its full meaning and discovers all the truth of which love is the human symbol, all its essential instincts divinised, raised, satisfied in the bliss from which our life was born and towards which by oneness it returns in the Ananda of the divine existence where love is absolute, eternal and unalloyed.

---

1. These are three of the four classes of devotee which are recognised by the Gita, *ārta*, *arthārthī*, *jijñāsu*, the distressed, the seeker of personal objects and the seeker of God-knowledge.

THE WAY OF DEVOTION

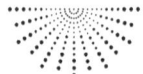

BHAKTI in itself is as wide as the heart-yearning of the soul for the Divine and as simple and straightforward as love and desire going straight towards their object. It cannot therefore be fixed down to any systematic method, cannot found itself on a psychological science like the Rajayoga, or a psycho-physical like the Hathayoga, or start from a definite intellectual process like the ordinary method of the Jnanayoga. It may employ various means or supports, and man, having in him a tendency towards order, process and system, may try to methodise his resort to these auxiliaries: but to give an account of their variations one would have to review almost all man's numberless religions upon their side of inner approach to the Deity. Really, however, the more intimate yoga of Bhakti resolves itself simply into these four movements, the desire of the Soul when it turns towards God and the straining of its emotion towards him, the pain of love and the divine return of love, the delight of love possessed and the play of that delight, and the eternal enjoyment of the divine Lover which is the heart of celestial bliss. These are things that are at once too simple and too profound for methodising or for analysis. One can at best only say, here are these four successive elements, steps, if we may so call them, of the siddhi, and here are, largely, some of the means which it uses, and here again are some of the aspects and experiences of the sadhana of devotion. We need only trace broadly the general line they follow before we turn to consider how the way of devotion enters into a synthetic and integral Yoga, what place it takes there and how its principle affects the other principles of divine living.

All Yoga is a turning of the human mind and the human soul, not yet divine in realisation, but feeling the divine impulse and attraction in it, towards that by which it finds its greater being. Emotionally, the first form which this turning takes must be that of adoration. In ordinary religion this adoration wears the form of external worship and that again develops a most external form of ceremonial worship. This element is ordinarily necessary because the mass of men live in their physical minds, cannot realise anything except by the force of a physical symbol and cannot feel that they are living anything except by the force of a physical action. We might apply here the Tantric gradation of *sādhana*, which makes the way of the *paśu*, the herd, the animal or physical being, the lowest stage of its discipline, and say that the purely or predominantly ceremonial adoration is the first step of this lowest part of the way. It is evident that even real religion, — and Yoga is something more than religion, — only begins when this quite outward worship corresponds to something really felt within the mind, some genuine submission, awe or spiritual aspiration, to which it becomes an aid, an outward expression and also a sort of periodical or constant reminder helping to draw back the mind to it from the preoccupations of ordinary life. But so long as it is only an idea of the Godhead to which one renders reverence or homage, we have not yet got to the beginning of Yoga. The aim of Yoga being union, its beginning must always be a seeking after the Divine, a longing after some kind of touch, closeness or possession. When this comes on us, the adoration becomes always primarily an inner worship; we begin to make ourselves a temple of the Divine, our thoughts and feelings a constant prayer of aspiration and seeking, our whole life an external service and worship. It is as this change, this new soul-tendency grows, that the religion of the devotee becomes a Yoga, a growing contact and union. It does not follow that the outward worship will necessarily be dispensed with, but it will increasingly become only a physical expression or outflowing of the inner devotion and adoration, the wave of the soul throwing itself out in speech and symbolic act.

Adoration, before it turns into an element of the deeper Yoga of devotion, a petal of the flower of love, its homage and self-uplifting to its sun, must bring with it, if it is profound, an increasing consecration of the being to the Divine who is adored.

And one element of this consecration must be a self-purifying so as to become fit for the divine contact, or for the entrance of the Divine into the temple of our inner being, or for his self-revelation in the shrine of the heart. This purifying may be ethical in its character, but it will not be merely the moralist's seeking for the right and blameless action or even, when once we reach the stage of Yoga, an obedience to the law of God as revealed in formal religion; but it will be a throwing away, *katharsis*, of all that conflicts whether with the idea of the Divine in himself or of the Divine in ourselves. In the former case it becomes in habit of feeling and outer act an imitation of the Divine, in the latter a growing into his likeness in our nature. What inner adoration is to ceremonial worship, this growing into the divine likeness is to the outward ethical life. It culminates in a sort of liberation by likeness to the Divine,[1] a liberation from our lower nature and a change into the divine nature.

Consecration becomes in its fullness a devoting of all our being to the Divine; therefore also of all our thoughts and our works. Here the Yoga takes into itself the essential elements of the Yoga of works and the Yoga of knowledge, but in its own manner and with its own peculiar spirit. It is a sacrifice of life and works to the Divine, but a sacrifice of love more than a tuning of the will to the divine Will. The bhakta offers up his life and all that he is and all that he has and all that he does to the Divine. This surrender may take the ascetic form, as when he leaves the ordinary life of men and devotes his days solely to prayer and praise and worship or to ecstatic meditation, gives up his personal possessions and becomes the monk or the mendicant whose one and only possession is the Divine, gives up all actions in life except those only which help or belong to the communion with the Divine and communion with other devotees, or at most keeps the doing from the secure fortress of the ascetic life of those services to men which seem peculiarly the outflowing of the divine nature of love, compassion and good. But there is the wider self-consecration, proper to any integral Yoga, which, accepting the fullness of life and the world in its entirety as the play of the Divine, offers up the whole being into his possession; it is a holding of all one is and has as belonging to him only and not to ourselves and a doing of all works as an offering to him. By this comes the complete active consecration of both the inner and the outer life, the unmutilated self-giving.

There is also the consecration of the thoughts to the Divine. In its inception this is the attempt to fix the mind on the object of adoration, — for naturally the restless human mind is occupied with other objects and, even when it is directed upwards, constantly drawn away by the world, — so that in the end it habitually thinks of him and all else is only secondary and thought of only in relation to him. This is done often with the aid of a physical image or, more intimately and characteristically, of a mantra or a divine name through which the divine being is realised. There are supposed by those who systematise to be three stages of the seeking through the devotion of the mind, first, the constant hearing of the divine name, qualities and all that has been attached to them, secondly, the constant thinking on them or on the divine being or personality, thirdly, the settling and fixing of the mind on the object; and by this comes the full realisation. And by these, too there comes when the accompanying feeling or the concentration is very intense, the Samadhi, the ecstatic trance in which the consciousness passes away from outer objects. But all this is really incidental; the one thing essential is the intense devotion of the thought in the mind to the object of adoration. Although it seems akin to the contemplation of the way of knowledge, it differs from that in its spirit. It is in its real nature not a still, but an ecstatic contemplation; it seeks not to pass into the being of the Divine, but to bring the Divine into ourselves and to lose ourselves in the deep ecstasy of his presence or of his possession; and its bliss is not the peace of unity, but the ecstasy of union. Here, too, there may be the separative self-consecration which ends in the giving up of all other thought of life for the possession of this ecstasy, eternal afterwards in planes beyond, or the comprehensive consecration in which all the thoughts are full of the Divine and even in the occupations of life every thought remembers him. As in the other Yogas, so in this, one comes to see the Divine everywhere and in all and to pour out the realisation of the Divine in all one's inner activities and outward actions. But all is supported here by the primary force of the emotional union: for it is by love that the entire self-consecration and the entire possession is accomplished, and thought and action become shapes and figures of the divine love which possesses the spirit and its members.

This is the ordinary movement by which what may be at first a vague adoration of some idea of the Divine takes on the hue and character and then, once entered into the path of Yoga, the inner reality and intense experience of divine love. But there is the more intimate Yoga which from the first consists in this love and attains only by the intensity of its longing without other process or method. All the rest comes, but it comes out of this, as leaf and flower out of the seed; other things are not the means of developing and fulfilling love, but the radiations of love already growing in the soul. This is the way that the soul follows when, while occupied perhaps with the normal human life, it has heard the flute of the Godhead behind the near screen of secret woodlands and no longer possesses itself, can have no satisfaction or rest till it has pursued and seized and possessed the divine fluteplayer. This is in essence the power of love itself in the heart and soul turning from earthly objects to the spiritual source of all beauty and delight. There live in this seeking all the sentiment and passion, all the moods and experiences of love concentrated on a supreme object of desire and intensified a hundredfold beyond the highest acme of intensity possible to a human love. There is the disturbance of the whole life, the illumination by an unseized vision, the unsatisfied yearning for a single object of the heart's desire, the intense impatience of all that distracts from the one preoccupation, the intense pain of the obstacles that stand in the way of possession, the perfect vision of all beauty and delight in a single form. And there are all the many moods of love, the joy of musing and absorption, the delight of the meeting and fulfilment and embrace, the pain of separation, the wrath of love, the tears of longing, the increased delight of reunion. The heart is the scene of this supreme idyll of the inner consciousness, but a heart which undergoes increasingly an intense spiritual change and becomes the radiantly unfolding lotus of the spirit. And as the intensity of its seeking is beyond the highest power of the normal human emotions, so also the delight and the final ecstasy are beyond the reach of the imagination and beyond expression by speech. For this is the delight of the Godhead that passes human understanding.

Indian bhakti has given to this divine love powerful forms, poetic symbols which are not in reality so much symbols as intimate expressions of truth which can find no other expression. It uses human relations and sees a divine person, not as mere figures, but because there are divine relations of supreme Delight and Beauty with the human soul of which human relations are the imperfect but still the real type, and because that Delight and Beauty are not abstractions or qualities of a quite impalpable metaphysical entity, but the very body and form of the supreme Being. It is a living Soul to which the soul of the bhakta yearns; for the source of all life is not an idea or a conception or a state of existence, but a real Being. Therefore in the possession of the divine Beloved all the life of the soul is satisfied and all the relations by which it finds and in which it expresses itself, are wholly fulfilled; therefore, too, by any and all of them can the Beloved be sought, though those which admit the greatest intensity, are always those by which he can be most intensely pursued and possessed with the profoundest ecstasy. He is sought within in the heart and therefore apart from all by an inward-gathered concentration of the being in the soul itself; but he is also seen and loved everywhere where he manifests his being. All the beauty and joy of existence is seen as his joy and beauty; he is embraced by the spirit in all beings; the ecstasy of love enjoyed pours itself out in a universal love; all existence becomes a radiation of its delight and even in its very appearances is transformed into something other than its outward appearance. The world itself is experienced as a play of the divine Delight, a Lila, and that in which the world loses itself is the heaven of beatitude of the eternal union.

---

1. *sādṛśya-mukti.*

THE DIVINE PERSONALITY

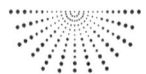

ONE QUESTION rises immediately in a synthetic Yoga which must not only comprise but unify knowledge and devotion, the difficult and troubling question of the divine Personality. All the trend of modern thought has been towards the belittling of personality; it has seen behind the complex facts of existence only a great impersonal force, an obscure becoming, and that too works itself out through impersonal forces and impersonal laws, while personality presents itself only as a subsequent, subordinate, partial, transient phenomenon upon the face of this impersonal movement. Granting even to this Force a consciousness, that seems to be impersonal, indeterminate, void in essence of all but abstract qualities or energies; for everything else is only a result, a minor phenomenon. Ancient Indian thought starting from quite the other end of the scale arrived on most of its lines at the same generalisation. It conceived of an impersonal existence as the original and eternal truth; personality is only an illusion or at best a phenomenon of the mind.

On the other hand, the way of devotion is impossible if the personality of the Divine cannot be taken as a reality, a real reality and not a hypostasis of the illusion. There can be no love without a lover and beloved. If our personality is an illusion and the Personality to whom our adoration rises only a primary aspect of the illusion, and if we believe that, then love and adoration must at once be killed, or can only survive in the illogical passion of the heart denying by its strong beats of life the clear and dry truths of the reason. To love and adore a shadow of our minds or a bright cosmic phenomenon which vanishes from the eye of Truth, may be possible, but the way of salvation cannot be built upon a foundation of wilful self-deception. The bhakta indeed does not allow these doubts of the intellect to come in his way; he has the divinations of his heart, and these are to him sufficient. But the sadhaka of the integral Yoga has to know the eternal and ultimate Truth and not to persist to the end in the delight of a Shadow. If the impersonal is the sole enduring truth, then a firm synthesis is impossible. He can at most take the divine personality as a symbol, a powerful and effective fiction, but he will have in the end to overpass it and to abandon devotion for the sole pursuit of the ultimate knowledge. He will have to empty being of all its symbols, values, contents in order to arrive at the featureless Reality.

We have said, however, that personality and impersonality, as our minds understand them, are only aspects of the Divine and both are contained in his being; they are one thing which we see from two opposite sides and into which we enter by two gates. We have to see this more clearly in order to rid ourselves of any doubts with which the intellect may seek to afflict us as we follow the impulse of devotion and the intuition of love or to pursue us into the joy of the divine union. They fall away indeed from that joy, but if we are too heavily weighted with the philosophical mind, they may follow us almost up to its threshold. It is well therefore to discharge ourselves of them as early as may be by perceiving the limits of the intellect, the rational philosophic mind, in its peculiar way of approaching the truth and the limits even of the spiritual experience which sets out from the approach through the intellect, to see that it need not be the whole integrality of the highest and widest spiritual experience. Spiritual intuition is always a more luminous guide than the discriminating reason, and spiritual intuition addresses itself to us not only through the reason, but through the rest of our being as well, through the heart and the life also. The integral knowledge will then be that which takes account of all and unifies their diverse truths. The intellect itself will be more deeply satisfied if it does not confine itself to its own data, but accepts truth of the heart and the life also and gives to them their absolute spiritual value.

The nature of the philosophical intellect is to move among ideas and to give them a sort of abstract reality of their own apart from all their concrete representations which affect our life and personal consciousness. Its bent is to reduce these representations to their barest and most general terms and to subtilise even these if possible into some final abstraction. The pure intellectual direction travels away from life. In judging things it tries to get back from their effects on our personality and to arrive at whatever general and impersonal truth may be behind them; it is inclined to treat that kind of truth as the only real truth of being or at least as the one superior and permanent power of reality. Therefore it is bound by its own nature to end in its extremes at an absolute impersonality and an absolute abstraction. This is where the ancient philosophies ended. They reduced everything to three abstractions, existence, consciousness and bliss of being, and they tended to get rid of the two of these three which seemed dependent on the first and most abstract, and to throw all back into a pure featureless existence from which everything else had been discharged, all representations, all values, except the one infinite and timeless fact of being. But the intellect had still one farther possible step to take and it took it in Buddhistic philosophy. It found that even this final fact of existence was only a representation; it abstracted that also and got to an infinite zero which might be either a void or an eternal inexpressible.

The heart and life, as we know, have an exactly opposite law. They cannot live with abstractions; they can find their satisfaction only in things that are concrete or can be made seizable; whether physically, mentally or spiritually, their object is not something which they seek to discriminate and arrive at by intellectual abstraction; a living becoming of it or a conscious possession and joy of their object is what they seek. Nor is it the satisfaction of an abstract mind or impersonal existence to which they respond, but the joy and the activity of a being, a conscious Person in us, whether finite or infinite, to whom the delights and powers of his existence are a reality. Therefore when the heart and life turn towards the Highest and the Infinite, they arrive not at an abstract existence or non-existence, a Sat or else a Nirvana, but at an existent, a Sat

Purusha, not merely at a consciousness, but at a conscious Being, a Chaitanya Purusha, not merely at a purely impersonal delight of the Is, but at an infinite I Am of bliss, an Anandamaya Purusha; nor can they immerge and lose his consciousness and bliss in featureless existence, but must insist on all three in one, for delight of existence is their highest power and without consciousness delight cannot be possessed. That is the sense of the supreme figure of the intensest Indian religion of love, Sri Krishna, the All-blissful and All-beautiful.

The intelligence can also follow this trend, but it ceases then to be the pure intellect; it calls in its power of imagination to its aid, it becomes the image-maker, the creator of symbols and values, a spiritual artist and poet. Therefore the severest intellectual philosophy admits the Saguna, the divine Person, only as the supreme cosmic symbol; go beyond it to reality and you will arrive, it says, at last to the Nirguna, the pure Impersonal. The rival philosophy asserts the superiority of the Saguna; that which is impersonal is, it will perhaps say, only the material, the stuff of his spiritual nature out of which he manifests the powers of his being, consciousness and bliss, all that expresses him; the impersonal is the apparent negative out of which he looses the temporal variations of his eternal positive of personality. There are evidently here two instincts, or, if we hesitate to apply that word to the intellect, two innate powers of our being which are dealing each in its own manner with the same Reality.

Both the ideas of the intellect, its discriminations, and the aspirations of the heart and life, their approximations, have behind them realities at which they are the means of arriving. Both are justified by spiritual experience; both arrive at the divine absolute of that which they are seeking. But still each tends, if too exclusively indulged, to be hampered by the limitations of its innate quality and its characteristic means. We see that in our earthly living, where the heart and life followed exclusively failed to lead to any luminous issue, while an exclusive intellectuality becomes either remote, abstract and impotent or a sterile critic or dry mechanist. Their sufficient harmony and just reconciliation is one of the great problems of our psychology and our action.

The reconciling power lies beyond in the intuition. But there is an intuition which serves the intellect and an intuition which serves the heart and the life, and if we follow either of these exclusively, we shall not get much farther than before; we shall only make more intimately real to us, but still separately, the things at which the other and less seeing powers are aiming. But the fact that it can lend itself impartially to all parts of our being, — for even the body has its intuitions, — shows that the intuition is not exclusive, but an integral truth-finder. We have to question the intuition of our whole being, not only separately in each part of it, nor in a sum of their findings, but beyond all these lower instruments, beyond even their first spiritual correspondents, by rising into the native home of the intuition which is the native home of the infinite and illimitable Truth, *ṛtasya sve dame*, where all existence discovers its unity. That is what the ancient Veda meant when it cried, "There is a firm truth hidden by truth (the eternal truth concealed by this other of which we have here these lower intuitions); there the ten hundred rays of light stand together; that is One." *ṛtena ṛtam apihitaṁ dhruvaṁ . . . daśa śatā saha tasthus, tad ekam.*

The spiritual intuition lays hold always upon the reality; it is the luminous harbinger of spiritual realisation or else its illuminative light; it sees that which the other powers of our being are labouring to explore; it gets at the firm truth of the abstract representations of the intellect and the phenomenal representations of the heart and life, a truth which is itself neither remotely abstract nor outwardly concrete, but something else for which these are only two sides of its psychological manifestation to us. What the intuition of our integral being perceives, when its members no longer dispute among themselves but are illumined from above, is that the whole of our being aims at the one reality. The impersonal is a truth, the personal too is a truth; they are the same truth seen from two sides of our psychological activity; neither by itself gives the total account of the Reality, and yet by either we can approach it.

Looked at from one side, it would seem as if an impersonal Thought were at work and created the fiction of the thinker for the convenience of its action, an impersonal Power at work creating the fiction of the doer, an impersonal existence in operation which uses the fiction of a personal being who has a conscious personality and a personal delight. Looked at from the other side, it is the thinker who expresses himself in thoughts which without him could not exist and our general notion of thought symbolises simply the power of the nature of the thinker; the Ishwara expresses himself by will and power and force; the Existent extends himself in all the forms integral and partial, direct, inverse and perverse of his existence, consciousness and bliss, and our abstract general notion of these things is only an intellectual representation of the triple power of his nature of being. All impersonality seems in its turn to become a fiction and existence in its every movement and its every particle nothing but the life, the consciousness, the power, the delight of the one and yet innumerable Personality, the infinite Godhead, the self-aware and self-unfolding Purusha. Both views are true, except that the idea of fiction, which is borrowed from our own intellectual processes, has to be exiled and each must be given its proper validity. The integral seeker has to see in this light that he can reach one and the same Reality on both lines, either successively or simultaneously, as if on two connected wheels travelling on parallel lines, but parallel lines which in defiance of intellectual logic but in obedience to their own inner truth of unity do meet in infinity.

We have to look at the divine Personality from this standpoint. When we speak of personality, we mean by it at first something limited, external and separative, and our idea of a personal God assumes the same imperfect character. Our personality is to us at first a separate creature, a limited mind, body, character which we conceive of as the person we are, a fixed quantity; for although in reality it is always changing, yet there is a sufficient element of stability to give a kind of practical justification to this notion of fixedness. We conceive of God as such a person, only without body, a separate person different from all others with a mind and character limited by certain qualities. At first in our primitive conceptions his deity is a thing of much inconstancy, freak and caprice, an enlarged edition of our human character; but afterwards we conceive of the divine nature of personality as a quite fixed quantity and we attribute to it those qualities alone which we regard as divine and ideal, while all the others are eliminated. This limitation compels us to account for all the rest by attributing them to a Devil, or by lending to man an original creative capacity for all that we consider evil, or else, when we perceive that this will not quite do, by erecting a power which we call Nature and attributing to that all the lower quality and mass of action for which we do not wish to make the Divine responsible. At a higher pitch the attribution of mind and character to God becomes less anthropomorphic and we regard him as an infinite Spirit, but still a separate person, a spirit with certain fixed divine qualities as his attributes. So are conceived the ideas of the divine Personality, the personal God which vary so much in various religions.

All this may seem at first sight to be an original anthropomorphism terminating in an intellectual notion of the Deity which is very much at variance with the actualities of the world as we see it. It is not surprising that the philosophical and sceptical mind should have found little difficulty in destroying it all intellectually, whether in the direction of the denial of a personal God and the assertion of an impersonal Force or Becoming or in that of an impersonal Being or an ineffable denial of existence with all the rest as only symbols of Maya or phenomenal truths of the Time-consciousness. But these are only the personifications of monotheism. Polytheistic religions, less exalted perhaps, but wider and more sensitive in their response to cosmic life, have felt that all in the cosmos has a divine origin; therefore they conceived of the existence of many divine personalities with a vague sense of an indefinable Divine behind, whose relations with the personal gods were not very clearly conceived. And in their more exoteric forms these gods were crudely anthropomorphic; but where the inner sense of spiritual things became clearer, the various godheads assumed the appearance of personalities of the one Divine, — that is the declared point of view of the ancient Veda. This Divine might be a supreme Being who manifests himself in various divine personalities or an impersonal existence which meets the human mind in these forms; or both views might be held simultaneously without any intellectual attempt to reconcile them, since both were felt to be true to spiritual experience.

If we subject these notions of the divine Personality to the discrimination of the intellect, we shall be inclined to reduce them, according to our bent, to fictions of the imagination or to psychological symbols, in any case, the response of our sensitive personality to something which is not this at all, but is purely impersonal. We may say that That is in reality the very opposite of our humanity and our personality and therefore in order to enter into relations with it we are impelled to set up these human fictions and these personal symbols so as to make it nearer to us. But we have to judge by spiritual experience, and in a total spiritual experience we shall find that these things are not fictions and symbols, but truths of divine being in their essence, however imperfect may have been our representations of them. Even our first idea of our own personality is not an absolute error, but only an incomplete and superficial view beset by many mental errors. Greater self-knowledge shows us that we are not fundamentally the particular formulation of form, powers, properties, qualities with a conscious I identifying itself with them, which we at first appear to be. That is only a temporary fact, though still a fact, of our partial being on the surface of our active consciousness. We find within an infinite being with the potentiality of all qualities, of infinite quality, *ananta-guṇa*, which can be combined in any number of possible ways, and each combination is a revelation of our being. For all this personality is the self-manifestation of a Person, that is to say of a being who is conscious of his manifestation.

But we see too that this being does not seem to be composed even of infinite quality, but has a status of his complex reality in which he seems to stand back from it and to become an indefinable conscious existence, *anirdeśyam*. Even consciousness seems to be drawn back and leave merely a timeless pure existence. And again even this pure self of our being seems at a certain pitch to deny its own reality, or to be a projection from a selfless[1] baseless unknowable, which we may conceive of either as a nameless somewhat, or as a Nihil. It is when we would fix upon this exclusively and forget all that it has withdrawn into itself that we speak of pure impersonality or the void Nihil as the highest truth. But a more integral vision shows us that it is the Person and the personality and all that it had manifested which has thus cast itself upward into its own unexpressed absolute. And if we carry up our heart as well as our reasoning mind to the Highest, we shall find that we can reach it through the absolute Person as well as through an absolute impersonality. But all this self-knowledge is only the type within ourselves of the corresponding truth of the Divine in his universality. There too we meet him in various forms of divine personality; in formulations of quality which variously express him to us in his nature; in infinite quality, the Ananta-guṇa; in the divine Person who expresses himself through infinite quality; in absolute impersonality, an absolute existence or an absolute nonexistence, which is yet all the time the unexpressed Absolute of this divine Person, this conscious Being who manifests himself through us and through the universe.

Even on the cosmic plane we are constantly approaching the Divine on either of these sides. We may think, feel and say that God is Truth, Justice, Righteousness, Power, Love, Delight, Beauty; we may see him as a universal force or as a universal consciousness. But this is only the abstract way of experience. As we ourselves are not merely a number of qualities or powers or a psychological quantity, but a being, a person who so expresses his nature, so is the Divine a Person, a conscious Being who thus expresses his nature to us. And we can adore him through different forms of this nature, a God of righteousness, a God of love and mercy, a God of peace and purity; but it is evident that there are other things in the divine nature which we have put outside the form of personality in which we are thus worshipping him. The courage of an unflinching spiritual vision and experience can meet him also in more severe or in terrible forms. None of these are all the Divinity; yet these forms of his personality are real truths of himself in which he meets us and seems to deal with us, as if the rest had been put away behind him. He is each separately and all altogether. He is Vishnu, Krishna, Kali; he reveals himself to us in humanity as the Christ personality or the Buddha personality. When we look beyond our first exclusively concentrated vision, we see behind Vishnu all the personality of Shiva and behind Shiva all the personality of Vishnu. He is the Ananta-guna, infinite quality and the infinite divine Personality whith manifests itself through it. Again he seems to withdraw into a pure spiritual impersonality or beyond all idea even of impersonal Self and to justify a spiritualised atheism or agnosticism; he becomes to the mind of man an indefinable, *anirdeśyam*. But out of this unknowable the conscious Being, the divine Person, who has manifested himself here, still speaks, "This too is I; even here beyond the view of mind, I am He, the Purushottama."

For beyond the divisions and contradictions of the intellect there is another light and there the vision of a truth reveals itself which we may thus try to express to ourselves intellectually. There all is one truth of all these truths; for there each is present and justified in all the rest. In that light our spiritual experience becomes united and integralised; no least hair's breadth of real division is left, no shade of superiority and inferiority remains between the seeking of the Impersonal and the adoration of the divine Personality, between the way of knowledge and the way of devotion.

---

1. *anātmyam anilayanam*. Taittiriya Upanishad.

THE DELIGHT OF THE DIVINE

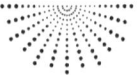

THIS THEN IS THE WAY OF DEVOTION and this its justification to the highest and the widest, the most integral knowledge, and we can now perceive what form and place it will take in an integral Yoga. Yoga is in essence the union of the soul with the immortal being and consciousness and delight of the Divine, effected through the human nature with a result of development into the divine nature of being, whatever that may be, so far as we can conceive it in mind and realise it in spiritual activity. Whatever we see of this Divine and fix our concentrated effort upon it, that we can become or grow into some kind of unity with it or at the lowest into tune and harmony with it. The old Upanishad put it trenchantly in its highest terms, "Whoever envisages it as the Existence becomes that existence and whoever envisages it as the Non-existence, becomes that non-existence;" so too it is with all else that we see of the Divine, — that, we may say, is at once the essential and the pragmatic truth of the Godhead. It is something beyond us which is indeed already within us, but which we as yet are not or are only initially in our human existence; but whatever of it we see, we can create or reveal in our conscious nature and being and can grow into it, and so to create or reveal in ourselves individually the Godhead and grow into its universality and transcendence is our spiritual destiny. Or if this seem too high for the weakness of our nature, then at least to approach, reflect and be in secure communion with it is a near and possible consummation.

The aim of this synthetic or integral Yoga which we are considering, is union with the being, consciousness and delight of the Divine through every part of our human nature separately or simultaneously, but all in the long end harmonised and unified, so that the whole may be transformed into a divine nature of being. Nothing less than this can satisfy the integral seer, because what he sees must be that which he strives to possess spiritually and, so far as may be, become. Not with the knower in him alone, nor with the will alone, nor with the heart alone, but with all these equally and also with the whole mental and vital being in him he aspires to the Godhead and labours to convert their nature into its divine equivalents. And since God meets us in many ways of his being and in all tempts us to him even while he seems to elude us, — and to see divine possibility and overcome its play of obstacles constitutes the whole mystery and greatness of human existence, — therefore in each of these ways at its highest or in the union of all, if we can find the key of their oneness, we shall aspire to track out and find and possess him. Since he withdraws into impersonality, we follow after his impersonal being and delight, but since he meets us also in our personality and through personal relations of the Divine with the human, that too we shall not deny ourselves; we shall admit both the play of the love and the delight and its ineffable union.

By knowledge we seek unity with the Divine in his conscious being: by works we seek also unity with the Divine in his conscious being, not statically, but dynamically, through conscious union with the divine Will; but by love we seek unity with him in all the delight of his being. For that reason the way of love, however narrow it may seem in some of its first movements, is in the end more imperatively all-embracing than any other motive of Yoga. The way of knowledge tends easily towards the impersonal and the absolute, may very soon become exclusive. It is true that it need not do so; since the conscious being of the Divine is universal and individual as well as transcendent and absolute, here too there may be and should be a tendency to integral realisation of unity and we can arrive by it at a spiritual oneness with God in man and God in the universe not less complete than any transcendent union. But still this is not quite imperative. For we may plead that there is a higher and a lower knowledge, a higher self-awareness and a lower self-awareness, and that here the apex of knowledge is to be pursued to the exclusion of the mass of knowledge, the way of exclusion preferred to the integral way. Or we may discover a theory of illusion to justify our rejection of all connection with our fellow-men and with the cosmic action. The way of works leads us to the Transcendent whose power of being manifests itself as a will in the world one in us and all, by identity with which we come, owing to the conditions of that identity, into union with him as the one self in all and as the universal self and Lord in the cosmos. And this might seem to impose a certain comprehensiveness in our realisation of the unity. But still this too is not quite imperative. For this motive also may lean towards an entire impersonality and, even if it leads to a continued participation in the activities of the universal Godhead, may be entirely detached and passive in its principle. It is only when delight intervenes that the motive of integral union becomes quite imperative.

This delight which is so entirely imperative, is the delight in the Divine for his own sake and for nothing else, for no cause or gain whatever beyond itself. It does not seek God for anything that he can give us or for any particular quality in him, but simply and purely because he is our self and our whole being and our all. It embraces the delight of the transcendence, not for the sake of transcendence, but because he is the transcendent; the delight of the universal, not for the sake of universality, but because he is the universal; the delight of the individual not for the sake of individual satisfaction, but because he is the individual. It goes behind all distinctions and appearances and makes no calculations of more or less in his being, but embraces him wherever he is and therefore everywhere, embraces him utterly in the seeming less as in the seeming more, in the apparent limitation as in the revelation of the illimitable; it has the intuition and the experience of his oneness and completeness everywhere. To seek after him for the sake of his absolute being alone is really to drive at our own individual gain, the gain of absolute peace. To possess him absolutely indeed is necessarily the aim of this delight in his being, but this comes when we possess him utterly and are utterly possessed by him and need be limited to no particular status or condition. To seek after him in some heaven of bliss is to seek him not for himself, but for the bliss of heaven; when we have all the true delight of his being, then heaven is within ourselves, and wherever he is and we are, there we have the joy of his kingdom. So too to seek him only in ourselves and for ourselves, is to limit both ourselves and our joy in him. The integral delight embraces him not only within our own individual being, but equally in all men and in all beings. And because in him we are one with all, it seeks him not only for ourselves, but for all our fellows. A perfect and complete delight in the Divine, perfect because pure and self-existent, complete because all-embracing as well as all-absorbing, is the meaning of the way of Bhakti for the seeker of the integral Yoga.

Once it is active in us, all other ways of Yoga convert themselves, as it were, to its law and find by it their own richest significance. This integral devotion of our being to God does not turn away from knowledge; the bhakta of this path is the God-lover who is also the God-knower, because by knowledge of his being comes the whole delight of his being; but it is in delight that knowledge fulfils itself, the knowledge of the transcendent in the delight of the Transcendent, the knowledge of the universal in the delight of the universal Godhead, the knowledge of the individual manifestation in the delight of God in the individual, the knowledge of the impersonal in the pure delight of his impersonal being, the knowledge of the personal in the full delight of his personality, the knowledge of his qualities and their play in the delight of the manifestation, the knowledge of the quality-less in the delight of his colourless existence and non-manifestation.

So too this God-lover will be the divine worker, not for the sake of works or for a self-regarding pleasure in action, but because in this way God expends the power of his being and in his powers and their signs we find him, because the divine Will in works is the outflowing of the Godhead in the delight of its power, of divine Being in the delight of divine Force. He will feel perfect joy in the works and acts of the Beloved, because in them too he finds the Beloved; he will himself do all works because through those works too the Lord of his being expresses his divine joy in him: when he works, he feels that he is expressing in act and power his oneness with that which he loves and adores; he feels the rapture of the will which he obeys and with which all the force of his being is blissfully identified. So too, again, this God-lover will seek after perfection, because perfection is the nature of the Divine and the more he grows into perfection, the more he feels the Beloved manifest in his natural being. Or he will simply grow in perfection like the blossoming of a flower because the Divine is in him and the joy of the Divine, and as that joy expands in him, soul and mind and life too expand naturally into their godhead. At the same time, because he feels the Divine in all, perfect within every limiting appearance, he will not have the sorrow of his imperfection.

Nor will the seeking of the Divine through life and the meeting of him in all the activities of his being and of the universal being be absent from the scope of his worship. All Nature and all life will be to him at once a revelation and a fine trysting-place. Intellectual and aesthetic and dynamic activities, science and philosophy and life, thought and art and action will assume for him a diviner sanction and a greater meaning. He will seek them because of his clear sight of the Divine through them and because of the delight of the Divine in them. He will not be indeed attached to their appearances, for attachment is an obstacle to the Ananda; but because he possesses that pure, powerful and perfect Ananda which obtains everything but is dependent on nothing, and because he finds in them the ways and acts and signs, the becomings and the symbols and images of the Beloved, he draws from them a rapture which the normal mind that pursues them for themselves cannot attain or even dream. All this and more becomes part of the integral way and its consummation.

The general power of Delight is love and the special mould which the joy of love takes is the vision of beauty. The Godlover is the universal lover and he embraces the All-blissful and All-beautiful. When universal love has seized on his heart, it is the decisive sign that the Divine has taken possession of him; and when he has the vision of the All-beautiful everywhere and can feel at all times the bliss of his embrace, that is the decisive sign that he has taken possession of the Divine. Union is the consummation of love, but it is this mutual possession that gives it at once the acme and the largest reach of its intensity. It is the foundation of oneness in ecstasy.

THE ANANDA BRAHMAN

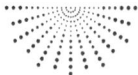

THE WAY OF DEVOTION in the integral synthetic Yoga will take the form of a seeking after the Divine through love and delight and a seizing with joy on all the ways of his being. It will find its acme in a perfect union of love and a perfect enjoyment of all the ways of the soul's intimacy with God. It may start from knowledge or it may start from works, but it will then turn knowledge into a joy of luminous union with the being of the Beloved and turn works into a joy of the active union of our being with the will and the power of being of the Beloved. Or it may start directly from love and delight; it will then take both these other things into itself and will develop them as part of the complete joy of oneness.

The beginning of the heart's attraction to the Divine may be impersonal, the touch of an impersonal joy in something universal or transcendent that has revealed itself directly or indirectly to our emotional or our aesthetic being or to our capacity of spiritual felicity. That which we thus grow aware of is the Ananda Brahman, the bliss existence. There is an adoration of an impersonal Delight and Beauty, of a pure and an infinite perfection to which we can give no name or form, a moved attraction of the soul to some ideal and infinite Presence, Power, existence in the world or beyond it, which in some way becomes psychologically or spiritually sensible to us and then more and more intimate and real. That is the call, the touch of the bliss existence upon us. Then to have always the joy and nearness of its presence, to know what it is, so as to satisfy the intellect and the intuitional mind of its constant reality, to put our passive and, so far as we can manage it, our active, our inner immortal and even our outer mortal being into perfect harmony with it, grow into a necessity of our living. And to open ourselves to it is what we feel to be the one true happiness, to live into it the sole real perfection.

A transcendent Bliss, unimaginable and inexpressible by the mind and speech, is the nature of the Ineffable. That broods immanent and secret in the whole universe and in everything in the universe. Its presence is described as a secret ether of the bliss of being, of which the Scripture says that, if this were not, none could for a moment breathe or live. And this spiritual bliss is here also in our hearts. It is hidden in from the toil of the surface mind which catches only at weak and flawed translations of it into various mental, vital and physical forms of the joy of existence. But if the mind has once grown sufficiently subtle and pure in its receptions and not limited by the grosser nature of our outward responses to existence, we can take a reflection of it which will wear perhaps wholly or predominantly the hue of whatever is strongest in our nature. It may present itself first as a yearning for some universal Beauty which we feel in Nature and man and in all that is around us; or we may have the intuition of some transcendent Beauty of which all apparent beauty here is only a symbol. That is how it may come to those in whom the aesthetic being is developed and insistent and the instincts which, when they find form of expression, make the poet and artist, are predominant. Or it may be the sense of a divine spirit of love or else a helpful and compassionate infinite Presence in the universe or behind or beyond it which responds to us when we turn the need of our spirit towards it. So it may first show itself when the emotional being is intensely developed. It may come near to us in other ways, but always as a Power or Presence of delight, beauty, love or peace which touches the mind, but is beyond the forms these things take ordinarily in the mind.

For all joy, beauty, love, peace, delight are outflowings from the Ananda Brahman, — all delight of the spirit, the intellect, the imagination, aesthetic sense, ethical aspiration and satisfaction, action, life, the body. And through all ways of our being the Divine can touch us and make use of them to awaken and liberate the spirit. But to reach the Ananda Brahman in itself the mental reception of it must be subtilised, spiritualised, universalised, discharged of everything that is turbid and limiting. For when we draw quite near or enter into it, it is by an awakened spiritual sense of a transcendent and a universal Delight which exists within and yet behind and beyond the contradictions of the world and to which we can unite ourselves through a growing universal and spiritual or a transcendental ecstasy.

Ordinarily, the mind is satisfied with reflecting this Infinity we perceive or with feeling the sense of it within and without us, as an experience which, however frequent, yet remains exceptional. It seems in itself so satisfying and wonderful when it comes and our ordinary mind and the active life which we have to lead may seem to us so incompatible with it, that we may think it excessive to expect anything more. But the very spirit of Yoga is this, to make the exceptional normal, and to turn that which is above us and greater than our normal selves into our own constant consciousness. Therefore we should not hesitate to open ourselves more steadily to whatever experience of the Infinite we have, to purify and intensify it, to make it our object of constant thought and contemplation, till it becomes the originating power that acts in us, the Godhead we adore and embrace, our whole being is put into tune with it and it is made the very self of our being.

Our experience of it has to be purified of any mental alloy in it, otherwise it departs, we cannot hold it. And part of this purification is that it shall cease to be dependent on any cause or exciting condition of mind; it must become its own cause and self-existent, source of all other delight, which will exist only by it, and not attached to any cosmic or other image or symbol through which we first came into contact with it. Our experience of it has to be constantly intensified and made more concentrated; otherwise we shall only reflect it in the mirror of the imperfect mind and not reach that point of uplifting and transfiguration by which we are carried beyond the mind into the ineffable bliss. Object of our constant thought and contemplation, it will turn all that is into itself, reveal itself as the universal Ananda Brahman and make all existence its outpouring. If we wait upon it for the inspiration of all our inner and our outer acts, it will become the joy of the Divine pouring itself through us in light and love and power on life and all that lives. Sought by the adoration and love of the soul, it reveals itself as the Godhead, we see in it the face of God and know the bliss of our Lover. Tuning our whole being to it, we grow into a happy perfection of likeness to it, a human rendering of the divine nature. And when it becomes in every way the self of our self, we are fulfilled in being and we bear the plenitude.

Brahman always reveals himself to us in three ways, within ourselves, above our plane, around us in the universe. Within us, there are two centres of the Purusha, the inner Soul through which he touches us to our awakening; there is the Purusha in the lotus of the heart which opens upward all our powers and the Purusha in the thousand-petalled lotus whence descend through the thought and will, opening the third eye in us, the lightnings of vision and the fire of the divine energy. The bliss existence may come to us through either one of these centres. When the lotus of the heart breaks open, we feel a divine joy, love and peace expanding in us like a flower of light which irradiates the whole being. They can then unite themselves with their secret source, the Divine in our hearts, and adore him as in a temple; they can flow upwards to take possession of the thought and the will and break out upward towards the Transcendent; they stream out in thought and feeling and act towards all that is around us. But so long as our normal being offers any obstacle or is not wholly moulded into a response to this divine influence or an instrument of this divine possession, the experience will be intermittent and we may fall back constantly into our old mortal heart; but by repetition, *abhyāsa*, or by the force of our desire and adoration of the Divine, it will be progressively remoulded until this abnormal experience becomes our natural consciousness.

When the other upper lotus opens, the whole mind becomes full of a divine light, joy and power, behind which is the Divine, the Lord of our being on his throne with our soul beside him or drawn inward into his rays; all the thought and will become then a luminosity, power and ecstasy; in communication with the Transcendent, this can pour down towards our mortal members and flow by them outwards on the world. In this dawn too there are, as the Vedic mystics knew, our alternations of its day and night, our exiles from the light; but as we grow in the power to hold this new existence, we become able to look long on the sun from which this irradiation proceeds and in our inner being we can grow one body with it. Sometimes the rapidity of this change depends on the strength of our longing for the Divine thus revealed, and on the intensity of our force of seeking; but at others it proceeds rather by a passive surrender to the rhythms of his all-wise working which acts always by its own at first inscrutable method. But the latter becomes the foundation when our love and trust are complete and our whole being lies in the clasp of a Power that is perfect love and wisdom.

The Divine reveals himself in the world around us when we look upon that with a spiritual desire of delight that seeks him in all things. There is often a sudden opening by which the veil of forms is itself turned into a revelation. A universal spiritual Presence, a universal peace, a universal infinite Delight has manifested, immanent, embracing, all-penetrating. This Presence by our love of it, our delight in it, our constant thought of it returns and grows upon us; it becomes the thing that we see and all else is only its habitation, form and symbol. Even all that is most outward, the body, the form, the sound, whatever our senses seize, are seen as this Presence; they cease to be physical and are changed into a substance of spirit. This transformation means a transformation of our own inner consciousness; we are taken by the surrounding Presence into itself and we become part of it. Our own mind, life, body become to us only its habitation and temple, a form of its working and an instrument of its self-expression. All is only soul and body of this delight.

This is the Divine seen around us and on our own physical plane. But he may reveal himself above. We see or feel him as a high-uplifted Presence, a great infinite of Ananda above us, — or in it, our Father in heaven, — and do not feel or see him in ourselves or around us. So long as we keep this vision, the mortality in us is quelled by that Immortality; it feels the light, power and joy and responds to it according to its capacity; or it feels the descent of the spirit and it is then for a time transformed or else uplifted into some lustre of reflection of the light and power; it becomes a vessel of the Ananda. But at other times it lapses into the old mortality and exists or works dully or pettily in the ruck of its earthly habits. The complete redemption comes by the descent of the divine Power into the human mind and body and the remoulding of their inner life into the divine image, — what the Vedic seers called the birth of the Son by the sacrifice. It is in fact by a continual sacrifice or offering, a sacrifice of adoration and aspiration, of works, of thought and knowledge, of the mounting flame of the Godward will that we build ourselves into the being of this Infinite.

When we possess firmly this consciousness of the Ananda Brahman in all of these three manifestations, above, within, around, we have the full oneness of it and embrace all existences in its delight, peace, joy and love; then all the worlds become the body of this self. But we have not the richest knowledge of this Ananda if it is only an impersonal presence, largeness or immanence that we feel, if our adoration has not been intimate enough for this Being to reveal to us out of its wide-extended joy the face and body and make us feel the hands of the Friend and Lover. Its impersonality is the blissful greatness of the Brahman, but from that can look out upon us the sweetness and intimate control of the divine Personality. For Ananda is the presence of the Self and Master of our being and the stream of its outflowing can be the pure joy of his Lila.

THE MYSTERY OF LOVE

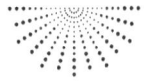

THE ADORATION of the impersonal Divine would not be strictly a Yoga of devotion according to the current interpretation; for in the current forms of Yoga it is supposed that the Impersonal can only be sought for a complete unity in which God and our own person disappear and there is none to adore or to be adored; only the delight of the experience of oneness and infinity remains. But in truth the miracles of spiritual consciousness are not to be subjected to so rigid a logic. When we first come to feel the presence of the infinite, as it is the finite personality in us which is touched by it, that may well answer to the touch and call with a sort of adoration. Secondly, we may regard the Infinite not so much as a spiritual status of oneness and bliss, or that only as its mould and medium of being, but rather as the presence of the ineffable Godhead to our consciousness, and then too love and adoration find their place. And even when our personality seems to disappear into unity with it, it may still be—and really is—the individual divine who is melting to the universal or the supreme by a union in which love and lover and loved are forgotten in a fusing experience of ecstasy, but are still there latent in the oneness and subconsciently persisting in it. All union of the self by love must necessarily be of this nature. We may even say, in a sense, that it is to have this joy of union as the ultimate crown of all the varied experiences of spiritual relation between the individual soul and God that the One became many in the universe.

Still, the more varied and most intimate experience of divine love cannot come by the pursuit of the impersonal Infinite alone; for that the Godhead we adore must become near and personal to us. It is possible for the Impersonal to reveal within itself all the riches of personality when we get into its heart, and one who sought only to enter into or to embrace the infinite Presence alone, may discover in it things he had not dreamed of; the being of the Divine has surprises for us which confound the ideas of the limiting intellect. But ordinarily the way of devotion begins from the other end; it starts from and it rises and widens to its issue by adoration of the divine Personality. The Divine is a Being and not an abstract existence or a status of pure timeless infinity; the original and universal existence is He, but that existence is inseparable from consciousness and bliss of being, and an existence conscious of its own being and its own bliss is what we may well call a divine infinite Person, — Purusha. Moreover all consciousness implies power, Shakti; where there is infinite consciousness of being, there is infinite power of being, and by that power all exists in the universe. All beings exist by this Being; all things are the faces of God; all thought and action and feeling and love proceed from him and return to him, all their results have him for source and support and secret goal. It is to this Godhead, this Being that the Bhakti of an integral Yoga will be poured out and uplifted. Transcendent, it will seek him in the ecstasy of an absolute union; universal, it will seek him in infinite quality and every aspect and in all beings with a universal delight and love; individual, it will enter into all human relations with him that love creates between person and person.

It may not be possible to seize from the beginning on all the complete integrality of that which the heart is seeking; in fact, it is only possible if the intelligence, the temperament, the emotional mind have already been developed into largeness and fineness by the trend of our previous living. That is what the experience of the normal life is meant to lead to by its widening culture of the intellect, the aesthetic and emotional mind and of our parts too of will and active experience. It widens and refines the normal being so that it may open easily to all the truth of That which was preparing it for the temple of its self-manifestation. Ordinarily, man is limited in all these parts of his being and he can grasp at first only so much of the divine truth as has some large correspondence to his own nature and its past development and associations. Therefore God meets us first in different limited affirmations of his divine qualities and nature; he presents himself to the seeker as an absolute of the things he can understand and to which his will and heart can respond; he discloses some name and aspect of his Godhead. This is what is called in Yoga the *iṣṭa-devatā*, the name and form elected by our nature for its worship. In order that the human being may embrace this Godhead with every part of himself, it is represented with a form that answers to its aspects and qualities and which becomes the living body of God to the adorer. These are those forms of Vishnu, Shiva, Krishna, Kali, Durga, Christ, Buddha, which the mind of man seizes on for adoration. Even the monotheist who worships a formless Godhead, yet gives to him some form of quality, some mental form or form of Nature by which he envisages and approaches him. But to be able to see a living form, a mental body, as it were, of the Divine gives to the approach a greater closeness and sweetness.

The way of the integral Yoga of bhakti will be to universalise this conception of the Deity, to personalise him intimately by a multiple and an all-embracing relation, to make him constantly present to all the being and to devote, give up, surrender the whole being to him, so that he shall dwell near to us and in us and we with him and in him. *Manana* and *darśana*, a constant thinking of him in all things and seeing of him always and everywhere is essential to this way of devotion. When we look on the things of physical Nature, in them we have to see the divine object of our love; when we look upon men and beings, we have to see him in them and in our relation with them to see that we are entering into relations with forms of him; when breaking beyond the limitation of the material world we know or have relations with the beings of other planes, still the same thought and vision has to be made real to our minds. The normal habit of our minds which are open only to the material and apparent form and the ordinary mutilated relation and ignore the secret Godhead within, has to yield by an unceasing habit of all-embracing love and delight to this deeper and ampler comprehension and this greater relation. In all godheads we have to see this one God whom we worship with our heart and all our being; they are forms of his divinity. So enlarging our spiritual embrace we reach a point at which all is he and the delight of this consciousness becomes to us our normal uninterrupted way of looking at the world. That brings us the outward or objective universality of our union with him.

Inwardly, the image of the Beloved has to become visible to the eye within, dwelling in us as in his mansion, informing our hearts with the sweetness of his presence, presiding over all our activities of mind and life as the friend, master and lover from the summit of our being, uniting us from above with himself in the universe. A constant inner communion is the joy to be made close and permanent and unfailing. This communion is not to be confined to an exceptional nearness and adoration when we retire quite into ourselves away from our normal preoccupations, nor is it to be sought by a putting away of our human activities. All our thoughts, impulses, feelings, actions have to be referred to him for his sanction or disallowance, or if we cannot yet reach this point, to be offered to him in our sacrifice of aspiration, so that he may more and more descend into us and be present in them all and pervade them with all his will and power, his light and knowledge, his love and delight. In the end all our thoughts, feelings, impulses, actions will begin to proceed from him and change into some divine seed and form of themselves; in our whole inner living we shall have grown conscious of ourselves as a part of his being till between the existence of the Divine whom we adore and our own lives there is no longer any division. So too in all happenings we have to come to see the dealings with us of the divine Lover and take such pleasure in them that even grief and suffering and physical pain become his gifts and turn to delight and disappear finally into delight, slain by the sense of the divine contact, because the touch of his hands is the alchemist of a miraculous transformation. Some reject life because it is tainted with grief and pain, but to the God-lover grief and pain become means of meeting with him, imprints of his pressure and finally cease as soon as our union with his nature becomes too complete for these masks of the universal delight at all to conceal it. They change into the Ananda.

All the relations by which this union comes about, become on this path intensely and blissfully personal. That which in the end contains, takes up or unifies them all, is the relation of lover and beloved, because that is the most intense and blissful of all and carries up all the rest into its heights and yet exceeds them. He is the teacher and guide and leads us to knowledge; at every step of the developing inner light and vision, we feel his touch like that of the artist moulding our clay of mind, his voice revealing the truth and its word, the thought he gives us to which we respond, the flashing of his spears of lightning which chase the darkness of our ignorance. Especially, in proportion as the partial lights of the mind become transformed into lights of gnosis, in whatever slighter or greater degree that may happen, we feel it as a transformation of our mentality into his and more and more he becomes the thinker and seer in us. We cease to think and see for ourselves, but think only what he wills to think for us and see only what he sees for us. And then the teacher is fulfilled in the lover; he lays hands on all our mental being to embrace and possess, to enjoy and use it.

He is the Master; but in this way of approach all distance and separation, all awe and fear and mere obedience disappear, because we become too close and united with him for these things to endure and it is the lover of our being who takes it up and occupies and uses and does with it whatever he wills. Obedience is the sign of the servant, but that is the lowest stage of this relation, *dāsya*. Afterwards we do not obey, but move to his will as the string replies to the finger of the musician. To be the instrument is this higher stage of self-surrender and submission. But this is the living and loving instrument and it ends in the whole nature of our being becoming the slave of God, rejoicing in his possession and its own blissful subjection to the divine grasp and mastery. With a passionate delight it does all he wills it to do without questioning and bears all he would have it bear, because what it bears is the burden of the beloved being.

He is the friend, the adviser, helper, saviour in trouble and distress, the defender from enemies, the hero who fights our battles for us or under whose shield we fight, the charioteer, the pilot of our ways. And here we come at once to a closer intimacy; he is the comrade and eternal companion, the playmate of the game of living. But still there is so far a certain division, however pleasant, and friendship is too much limited by the appearance of beneficence. The lover can wound, abandon, be wroth with us, seem to betray, yet our love endures and even grows by these oppositions; they increase the joy of reunion and the joy of possession; through them the lover remains the friend, and all that he does we find in the end has been done by the lover and helper of our being for our soul's perfection as well as for his joy in us. These contradictions lead to a greater intimacy. He is the father and mother too of our being, its source and protector and its indulgent cherisher and giver of our desires. He is the child born to our desire whom we cherish and rear. All these things the lover takes up; his love in its intimacy and oneness keeps in it the paternal and maternal care and lends itself to our demands upon it. All is unified in that deepest many-sided relation.

From the beginning even it is possible to have this closest relation of the lover and beloved, but it will not be as exclusive for the integral Yogin as for certain purely ecstatic ways of Bhakti. It will from the beginning take into itself something of the hues of the other relations, since he follows too knowledge and works and has need of the Divine as teacher, friend and master. The growing of the love of God must carry with it in him an expansion of the knowledge of God and of the action of the divine Will in his nature and living. The divine Lover reveals himself; he takes possession of the life. But still the essential relation will be that of love from which all things flow, love passionate, complete, seeking a hundred ways of fulfilment, every means of mutual possession, a million facets of the joy of union. All the distinctions of the mind, all its barriers and "cannot be"s, all the cold analyses of the reason are mocked at by this love or they are only used as the tests and fields and gates of union. Love comes to us in many ways; it may come as an awakening to the beauty of the Lover, by the sight of an ideal face and image of him, by his mysterious hints to us of himself behind the thousand faces of things in the world, by a slow or sudden need of the heart, by a vague thirst in the soul, by the sense of someone near us drawing us or pursuing us with love or of someone blissful and beautiful whom we must discover.

We may seek after him passionately and pursue the unseen beloved; but also the lover whom we think not of, may pursue us, may come upon us in the midst of the world and seize on us for his own whether at first we will or no. Even, he may come to us at first as an enemy, with the wrath of love, and our earliest relations with him may be those of battle and struggle. Where first there is love and attraction, the relations between the Divine and the soul may still for long be chequered with misunderstanding and offence, jealousy and wrath, strife and the quarrels of love, hope and despair and the pain of absence and separation. We throw up all the passions of the heart against him, till they are purified into a sole ecstasy of bliss and oneness. But that too is no monotony; it is not possible for the tongue of human speech to tell all the utter unity and all the eternal variety of the ananda of divine love. Our higher and our lower members are both flooded with it, the mind and life no less than the soul: even the physical body takes its share of the joy, feels the touch, is filled in all its limbs, veins, nerves with the flowing of the wine of the ecstasy, *amṛta*. Love and Ananda are the last word of being, the secret of secrets, the mystery of Mysteries.

Thus universalised, personalised, raised to its intensities, made all-occupying, all-embracing, all-fulfilling, the way of love and delight gives the supreme liberation. Its highest crest is a supracosmic union. But for love complete union is *mukti*; liberation has to it no other sense; and it includes all kinds of *mukti* together, nor are they in the end, as some would have it, merely successive to each other and therefore mutually exclusive. We have the absolute union of the divine with the human spirit, *sāyujya*; in that reveals itself a content of all that depends here upon difference, — but there the difference is only a form of oneness, — ananda too of nearness and contact and mutual presence, *sāmīpya*, *sālokya*, ananda of mutual reflection, the thing that we call likeness, *sādṛśya*, and other wonderful things too for which language has as yet no name. There is nothing which is beyond the reach of the God-lover or denied to him; for he is the favourite of the divine Lover and the self of the Beloved.

ALSO BY SRI AUROBINDO

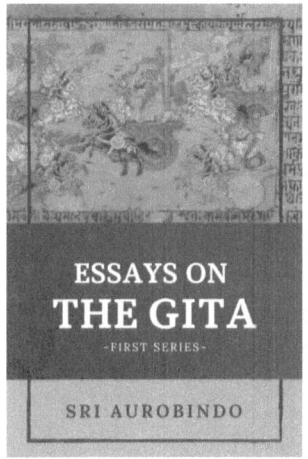

ESSAYS ON THE GITA

FIRST SERIES

- ISBN PAPERBACK: 9782357286313
- ISBN HARDCOVER: 9782357286320
- ISBN E-BOOK: 9782357286337

SECOND SERIES

- ISBN PAPERBACK: 9782357286481
- ISBN HARDCOVER: 9782357286498
- ISBN E-BOOK: 9782357286504

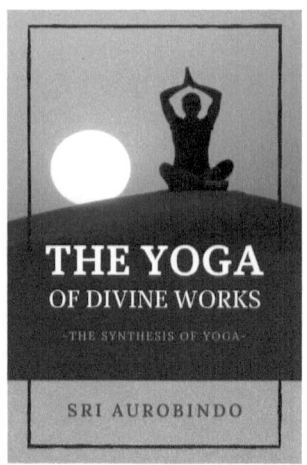

THE YOGA OF DIVINE WORKS

- ISBN PAPERBACK: 9782357286511
- ISBN HARDCOVER: 9782357286528
- ISBN E-BOOK: 9782357286535

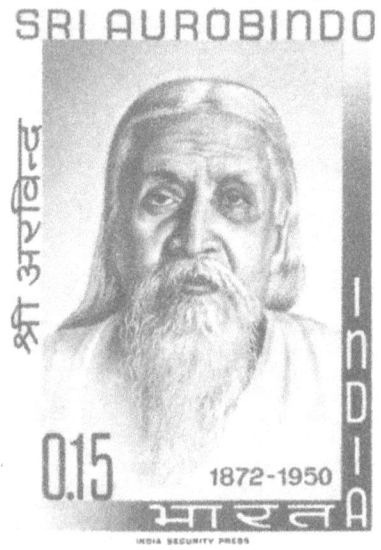

Copyright © 2020 by ALICIA EDITIONS
Credits: Canva
All rights reserved.
No part of this book may be reproduced in any form or by any electronic or mechanical means, including information storage and retrieval systems, without written permission from the author, except for the use of brief quotations in a book review.

www.ingramcontent.com/pod-product-compliance
Lightning Source LLC
LaVergne TN
LVHW040155080526
838202LV00042B/3171